WOMEN LIVING WITH FIBROMYALGIA

▲▲▲

Praise for Mari Skelly's previous book, *Alternative Treatments for Fibromyalgia & Chronic Fatigue Syndrome*

"Knowledge is power and the best tool to help ourselves. Thank you, Mari Skelly ... for bringing this much needed publication into light."
— Tracy S. Swenson, MS, PT, LMT; *Book Review.com*

"[A] helpful book for FM & CFS ... [that] addresses the wide range of alternative approaches to these two conditions."
— *New Living Magazine*

"This book is very informative about the wide spectrum of treatments available. You have to educate yourself as much as possible [about FM or CFS].... This is a very valuable book along those lines."
— Eduardo Barrera, owner, GravityWerks (quoted from *West Seattle Herald*)

"This book is a helpful aid for individuals who want to hear what others with fibromyalgia or CFS have to say about their experiences. [Mari Skelly takes] a sensible, balanced approach to treatment, and notes that although the book focuses predominantly on alternative therapies, readers should consider the full range of options available."
— Renee Brehio, *CFIDS Chronicle*

"[This book offers] an excellent range of treatment alternatives ... complete with detailed interviews with treatment experts who explain how each therapy works and what it does to help you."
— *ImmuneSupport.com*

Ordering

Trade bookstores in the U.S. and Canada please contact:

Publishers Group West
1700 Fourth Street, Berkeley CA 94710
Phone: (800) 788-3123   Fax: (510) 528-3444

Hunter House books are available at bulk discounts for textbook course adoptions; to qualifying community, health-care, and government organizations; and for special promotions and fund-raising. For details please contact:

Special Sales Department
Hunter House Inc., PO Box 2914, Alameda CA 94501-0914
Phone: (510) 865-5282   Fax: (510) 865-4295
E-mail: ordering@hunterhouse.com

Individuals can order our books from most bookstores, by calling
(800) 266-5592, or from our website at www.hunterhouse.com

Women Living with Fibromyalgia

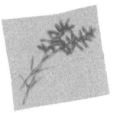

Mari Skelly

with Kelley Blewster

FOREWORD BY DEVIN J. STARLANYL

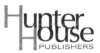

Hunter House Inc., Publishers
PO Box 2914
Alameda CA 94501-0914

Library of Congress Cataloging-in-Publication Data

Skelly, Mari.
Women living with fibromyalgia / Mari Skelly, with Kelley Blewster
p. cm.
Includes index.
ISBN 0-89793-343-5 (cl) — ISBN 0-89793-342-7 (pb)
1. Fibromyalgia—Popular works. 2. Women—Diseases—Popular works. I. Title.
RC927.3 .K43 2001
616.7'42'0082—dc21   2001026469

Project Credits

Cover Design: Suellen Ehnebuske, Jil Weil
Book Production: Hunter House
Developmental and Copy Editor: Kelley Blewster
Proofreader: David Marion
Indexer: Nancy D. Peterson
Acquisitions Editor: Jeanne Brondino
Editor: Alexandra Mummery
Publicity Coordinator: Earlita K. Chenault
Sales & Marketing Coordinator: JoAnne Retzlaff
Customer Service Manager: Christina Sverdrup
Order Fulfillment: Lakdhon Lama
Administrator: Theresa Nelson
Computer Support: Peter Eichelberger
Publisher: Kiran S. Rana

Printed and Bound by Transcontinental Printing in Canada

9 8 7 6 5 4 3 2 1   First Edition   02 03 04 05 06

Contents

Foreword

by DEVIN J. STARLANYL

You are about to invite some very special people into your life. As you read their words, you will see some of your own story reflected. Fibromyalgia (FM) syndrome isn't *curable* at this moment, but it is very *treatable*. Creating a new life while coping with FM is an ever-evolving process. This book is a collection of snapshots showing you how some women deal with that process.

Many years ago I created the word "FMily" to express the bond shared by those of us with FM. We live with a bewildering set of symptoms that can vary from hour to hour and day to day. Each of us has different neurotransmitters, hormones, and other biochemicals out of balance, requiring that each treatment plan be developed on a personal basis. This is time-consuming and difficult for doctors and patients alike.

Our society often places a stigma on people with chronic, invisible illnesses. An astounding number of caregivers "don't believe in" FM, in spite of the enormous amount of medical research showing that it is very real and life-altering. One study found that "the most aggressive challenges of the FMS concept have been from legal defenses of insurance carriers motivated by economic concerns. Other forms of critique have presented as psychiatric dogma, uninformed posturing, suspicion of malingering, ignorance of nociceptive physiology, and occasionally have resulted from honest misunderstanding."[1] Disbelief further burdens the patients, often denying them the support, respect, and medical care they deserve and desperately need.

Fibromyalgia is not a musculoskeletal illness; it is neurological.[2] It is not psychiatric in origin, and it should not be treated as such.[3,4] In FM, there is a generalized disturbance of how pain is processed. As the central nervous system becomes more sensitized, pain becomes more intense in response to any given stimulus, and this pain does not diminish as quickly as it does in a healthy individual. Eventually, the pain remains long after the stimulus or cause has ended. The FM patient feels amplified pain, and also may experience sensations of pain in response to normally nonpainful stimuli such as noise, touch, and light. The cognitive dysfunction that may also accompany FM can massively disrupt the patient's lifestyle. You keep losing things, and you begin to think that one of them is your mind. The world has become a game where the rules change daily, and nobody tells you what they are. You can easily become overwhelmed.

Parts of this book spoke to me of an urgent need for further education. Many symptoms these women describe are not part of FM syndrome at all. Ringing in the ears, numbness and tingling, specific muscle weakness, pelvic pain, pain during intercourse, failure of grip, lightning-like stabbing pain, knots and ropy bands in the muscles, foot pain, and hip pain are usually symptoms of myofascial trigger points (TrPs). *There are no trigger points in fibromyalgia!* Chronic myofascial pain due to TrPs is a separate but often coexisting condition.[5] Trigger points can be bodywide, and they can mimic FM, but they must be treated very differently.[6] For example, if a patient has only fibromyalgia, the muscles can be strengthened. By contrast, a muscle that is weak due to myofascial TrPs cannot be strengthened. The TrPs must be treated first. To optimally treat the pain *amplification* of FM, you must treat the pain *generators* such as TrPs.[7]

If someone with FM is getting steadily worse, that indicates the presence of one or more perpetuating factors that are not under control. Perpetuating factors—for example, sleep disturbance—cause a person's symptoms to remain in spite of appropriate treatment. She must obtain adequate, restorative sleep. When she wakes up she must feel refreshed. Sleep habits, diet, and other influences, as well as adequate medication, must be explored to optimize sleep. Pain, often the most important perpetuating factor, *must* be brought under control, because pain further stimulates the already oversensitized central nervous system of an FM patient. It can also worsen other perpetuating factors, such as sleep disruption and disturbance of gait. Yet many patients are denied adequate pain relief, which must include adequate medication and the identification and control of factors that may be contributing to pain. An FM patient may need to make lifestyle changes, such as quitting smoking, adding exercise, modifying her diet, and adding stress-reducing techniques. The latter may include, at least temporarily, removing a relative, job, or other stressor from her life. There are many possible neuroendocrine imbalances in FM. Prescribing a pill and recommending over-the-counter sleep aids does not constitute adequate medical care. Yet that is all many patients get, and some get even less. Those patients who have adequately educated physicians still need to marshal all of their support systems and strategies to cope with this time-consuming illness in which even a change in weather can exacerbate one's limitations.

In *Women Living with Fibromyalgia*, Mari Skelly has artfully woven the stories of a number of women into a colorful tapestry. Seeing the world through their eyes took me through a whirlwind of emotions. Each woman is a survivor on a tough road, and each has something of value to teach us. Mary started gathering her story threads with a detailed questionnaire, reproduced in the book at the end of Chapter 2. You may find it helpful to answer those questions yourself. If you have not been keeping a journal, this exercise could provide an excellent start.

These women are part of our FMily. You will learn how they deal with many challenges: relatives who don't understand, the loss or change of roles at work and at home, obtaining medications, handling financial challenges, fluctuating family dynamics, and dealing with the problems of intimacy brought on by chronic pain. As you read this book, pause from time to time to consider the difference between an obstacle and a challenge, both in their lives and yours. You will often find that the difference lies in attitude. It is not the stressors in our lives per se that cause havoc, but rather our reactions to them. Research shows that some patients with FM experience positive transformations.[8] As Mari Skelly has written, you are your own best advocate. There is life beyond FM, and you can live that life. This book will help you understand why I say that I have FM and myofascial TrPs, but they do not have me.

Devin J. Starlanyl is the author of Fibromyalgia and Chronic Myofascial Pain: A Survival Manual, *2nd edition (with Mary Ellen Copeland);* The Fibromyalgia Advocate; Chronic Myofascial Pain Syndrome: A Guide to the Trigger Points *(video);* Worlds of Power, Lines of Light *(FM science fiction); and the informational website www.sover.net/~devstar.*

References

1. Rau, C. L., Russell, I. J., 2000, "Is Fibromyalgia a Distinct Clinical Syndrome?" *Current Review of Pain* 4(4): 287–94.

2. Bradley, L. A., McKendree-Smith, N. L., Alarcon, G. S., et al., 2002, "Is Fibromyalgia a Neurologic Disease?" *Current Pain and Headache Reports* 6(2): 106–14.

3. Goldenberg, D. L., 1989, "Psychological Symptoms and Psychiatric Diagnosis in Patients with Fibromyalgia," *Journal of Rheumatology*, supplement, 19: 127–30.

4. Dunne, F. J., Dunne, C. A., 1995, "Fibromyalgia Syndrome and Psychiatric Disorder," *British Journal of Hospital Medicine* 54(5): 194–97.

5. Gerwin, R. D., 1999, "Differential Diagnosis of Myofascial Pain Syndrome and Fibromyalgia," *Journal of Musculoskeletal Pain* 7(1–2): 209–15.

6. Meyer, H. P., 2002, "Myofascial Pain Syndrome and Its Suggested Role in the Pathogenesis and Treatment of Fibromyalgia Syndrome," *Current Pain and Headache Reports* 6(4): 274–83.

7. Borg-Stein, J., 2002, "Management of Peripheral Pain Generators in Fibromyalgia," *Rheumatic Diseases Clinics of North America* 28(2): 305–17.

8. Asbring, P. J., 2001, "Chronic Illness—A Disruption in Life: Identity Transformation among Women with Chronic Fatigue Syndrome and Fibromyalgia," *Journal of Advanced Nursing* 34(3): 312–19.

IMPORTANT NOTE

The material in this book is intended to provide a review of information regarding fibromyalgia. Every effort has been made to provide accurate and dependable information. The contents of this book have been compiled through professional research and in consultation with medical professionals. However, health-care professionals have differing opinions, and advances in medical and scientific research are made very quickly, so some of the information may become outdated.

Therefore, the publisher, authors, and editors, and the professionals quoted in the book cannot be held responsible for any error, omission, or dated material. The authors and publisher assume no responsibility for any outcome of applying the information in this book in a program of self-care or under the care of a licensed practitioner. If you have questions concerning nutrition or your diet, or about the application of the information described in this book, consult a qualified health-care professional.

Introduction

I have spent the last five years talking to people about fibromyalgia (FM). It is a gift to hear about their everyday lives, their families, even their endless battles with pain and fatigue. They amaze me, these incredibly strong women, and they help me to manage my own life with FM. It is harder to shirk my exercise program when I have been telling people how important it is to stretch and to walk as much as they comfortably can.

After the 1999 publication of my first book, *Alternative Treatments for Fibromyalgia and Chronic Fatigue Syndrome* (ATF), I said to myself, "Working on this book was great, but boy, was it tough!" I spent the year after publication promoting the book by speaking to support groups, hospital groups, folks in bookstores, and people online. I think the excitement kept me going. Folks loved reading about the people in the book, and they saw themselves in the book. In every way, the best part about writing ATF was meeting such a wide range of people.

Then, in 2000, I crashed. I only gave a couple of online interviews that year. (I also gave away most of my personal copies of the book. It seemed that I met many people who were waiting for their Social Security benefits to be approved and for whom $15.95 was hard to come by.) I experienced a flare-up that reached epic proportions, with fatigue and pain I could find no relief from. Still, I pushed myself, because work in any form, if only for a few hours per week, is seductive. It pulls you back into the memory of who you were before becoming ill. Keeping life in balance takes hard work, and in 2000, I lost my balance. I even tried working a few hours a week at my old job as a florist. Why I thought I could stand in one spot (very difficult to do when you have tarsal tunnel syndrome, as I do) and design floral arrangements is a question I can't answer. I guess it was just my way of remembering my old life.

I have lived with FM for nine years. Let's just write off the first three years. They were spent desperately trying to understand how a healthy woman—who could easily work twelve-hour days at her job and then go home and work in her garden—could get so sick. I was thirty years old, jobless, and disabled, with an income of $333.00 per month. (Looking back now, I see how lucky I was. Some of the hundreds of women I have spoken to have lost their homes and their partners and have attempted suicide.) I became very scared and depressed.

My partner and I needed my income. We had just purchased a home and had been together for only two years. But, most important, I needed my job! I lived it. It was how I'd identified myself: Mari the Florist. Early on, I couldn't imagine how I could find joy in my day again. From there, working on ATF became a goal. If I could finish the book, I could prove to myself that there was life after FM. The key came when I realized my life wasn't over; it would now just be a different life.

A NEW KIND OF LIFE

In *The Pain Cure*, by Dharma Singh Khalsa, M.D., he tells us that pain and suffering do not go hand in hand. I believe this when I hear women such as Linda T. tell me, "I don't want this illness to get in the way of my living." In *Women Living with Fibromyalgia*, you will meet others like Linda: women who cope with FM in a proactive way. The book is constructed primarily of the frank testimonies of such women, most of whom have lived with FM for at least two years. Interwoven with the women's stories are my own experiences, as well as useful information about the illness and ways of dealing with it. Commentary from medical professionals is also included in a few chapters. But this book isn't centered around what the "professionals" have to say. Its purpose is to bring together and give voice to the experts in *living* with fibromyalgia.

Women Living with Fibromyalgia offers the reader many views on the myriad ways devised by women of living creatively with FM. Why women? Because women are diagnosed with this condition seven to ten times more often than men. When researching the book, I looked for women who worked, went to school, or had children. I knew that to lead such full lives, they must have tips they could share about how to cope with FM. But the book is more than a collection of "lemons from lemonade" tales. It doesn't sugarcoat the challenges of living with a debilitating chronic illness. You will also read passionate expressions of loss and grief. My hope is that wherever you are on the spectrum of learning to live with fibromyalgia, you will encounter someone in this book whose story of her physical, emotional, or spiritual experience resonates with yours.

I started the interview process by asking potential participants to complete a long essay questionnaire. The thirty-six questions ranged in topic from feelings about losing friends to finding help with pain management, from experiences with doctors to facing the daily crush of pain and fatigue. I feel fortunate to have been given the opportunity to hear the stories of the dozens of women I interviewed and to get to know them intimately. They have told me about their lives before and after the onset of FM, their losses, and, finally, their acceptance of a new kind of life. I have learned humorous and practical ways to get through the really bad times from women whose lives look a lot like mine.

You will meet these women up close in Chapter 2, which includes brief biographical sketches of all the participants, as well as the survey they responded to. But first, Chapter 1 attempts to answer the question "What is fibromyalgia?" There, you'll also encounter the first of the women's testimonies. Chapter 3 deals with women's reactions to finally receiving a diagnosis of fibromyalgia—often after many visits to doctors and months or years of confusion about what in the world was happening to our bodies. Chapter 4 takes a look at how FM affects women in particular—our menstrual cycles and other aspects of our health, our sexuality, our roles in our families and in the world.

Chapter 5 discusses treatment options, including pharmaceutical drugs, "alternative" or complementary therapies, and the roles played by diet and exercise. Chapter 6 covers emotional health—how to deal with the grief, anger, and isolation that almost invariably accompany the onset of a debilitating chronic illness such as FM. Chapter 7, "Everyday Solutions and Things That Really Work," as its title indicates, is full of practical ideas for helping you get through your day; it offers suggestions for managing your routine, as well as creative solutions for coping with three of FM's trademark symptoms: pain, fatigue, and "brain fog." Chapter 8 addresses one of the most challenging aspects of FM: dealing with loved ones and friends.

As consumers of medical care, we have rights and responsibilities. Chapter 9 looks at how our awareness of this fact affects our relationships with health-care providers, and also offers pointers on finding good doctors. Chapter 10, "Dealing with the Rest of the World," discusses expectations placed on us by society and by ourselves. A primary topic of the chapter is our changing relationship to our work and our careers. Chapter 11 addresses financial issues, especially the often-complicated process of claiming the Social Security benefits we're entitled to. In Chapter 12, "What's New? What's Coming?," I let a few medical professionals do most of the talking. They discuss advances in pharmaceutical treatment of fibromyalgia, some of the latest scientific research, and a couple of exciting new "alternative" treatments of FM.

A theme you'll encounter throughout this book is how women who live with fibromyalgia have created new, rewarding lives for themselves, even as they've grieved the passing of their old lives. Chapter 13 is devoted to this topic; in it we hear from our community of women about their lives and goals beyond FM, about the spiritual growth they've undergone in the face of the illness, and about other surprising, positive changes they've experienced from living with FM.

Women Living with Fibromyalgia brings together the voices of women from all over the United States (plus one from Australia). The result is a deep and thorough look into the lives of students, mothers, and professionals—retired and otherwise—living with fibromyalgia. They have much to teach us. Of all the people I have met during the process of compiling the material for the book, one woman stands out. I think about her a lot. I met her last year during an online interview. She is from a tiny town, and she said her doctor "didn't believe in FM." There were no support groups in her area, not even at the local hospital. She had no people in her life who understood the frustration of living with an invisible syndrome. She was unsure how to handle the ups and downs of FM. Her family failed to understand how she could look so good and yet say that she was exhausted and in extreme pain.

The reason her story sticks in my mind is because I have it so good here in my town and in my home. I live in Seattle, which is known countrywide as one of the best places for fibromyalgia support. I have a great rheumatologist. I have a partner who helps me out when I need it and friends who understand. My brother expressed concern about my well-being the other day. I thank God for all of these things, and more. Gifts can come in unexpected packages, as I've learned while living my new life since becoming ill.

SHARE YOUR STORY

For possible use in future writing projects, I invite you to send me your story of living with fibromyalgia—or any other comments or feedback you wish to share. Send it by e-mail to:
    fmcfsbook@earthlink.net

Or you can send it by U.S. mail to:
    Mari Skelly
    c/o Hunter House Publishers
    PO Box 2914, Alameda CA 94501-0914

I hope to hear from you!

What Is Fibromyalgia?

Before you officially meet the women whose stories form the foundation of the book, here are some basics about fibromyalgia: what are its symptoms, how is it diagnosed, and what is it like to live with the illness?

HOW DOES IT FEEL?

Fibromyalgia brings on pain like no other you have felt before—burning and aching in the muscles; sharp, stabbing pain in the tender points and elsewhere (see below for more about tender points); dull pain in the joints; and headache. It feels a lot like having the flu—for months or years at a time. For some FM patients, the allover flulike ache is constant. For others, it comes and goes.

In addition to the pain, there's the constant fatigue—even if you've slept the night before. Sleep is elusive and nonrestorative. The women in this book report having a hard time falling asleep and staying asleep. Many individuals with FM also endure a phenomenon called *restless-legs syndrome*, in which one's legs kick and move all night long, seemingly with a mind of their own.

Most people with FM report feeling very stiff in the morning. The morning stiffness seems to go away with a hot shower and movement.

Does all this sound familiar? You may be one of the up to ten million people in the United States who have fibromyalgia. Numbers differ depending on each book or newsletter, but all the statistics are staggering. Women are diagnosed with FM seven to ten times more often than men.

DIAGNOSIS

In 1990, the American College of Rheumatology established the following diagnostic criteria for fibromyalgia:

◀ Widespread pain lasting at least three months and existing in all four quadrants of the body (i.e., on both sides of the body and above and below the waist)

◀ Pain in at least eleven out of eighteen tender-point sites

Tender points are specific bodily sites that are painful to the touch. If one tender point is painful, so typically is its mate on the other side of the body. The tender-point sites include the top of the head (occipital region), the neck (lower cervical area), the area around the third rib, the upper back, the shoulder blades, the elbows, the top of the thigh, the buttocks, and the knees. When a health-care practitioner presses on a tender point of someone with fibromyalgia, the pressure creates intense pain of a sort that is different from the bodywide sensation of diffuse pain.

Right now, there is no single laboratory test to determine if you have FM. And pain, of course, is subjective. Many women who responded to my survey said that their doctors first ruled out such other conditions as lupus and multiple sclerosis before a diagnosis of FM was made.

OTHER SYMPTOMS

FM involves more than pain and fatigue. Some patients report headaches of a type different from the fairly common muscle-tension headache. Many FM patients also suffer migraines and temporomandibular joint syndrome (TMJS), a dysfunction that causes grinding and clicking in the temporomandibular joint, located where the temporal bone of the skull connects to the lower jaw (mandible). TMJS can also cause pain in the ears, face, and head.

Irritable bowel syndrome (IBS) and irritable bladder are two more common complaints among FM patients. Irritable bowel can cause diarrhea one day and constipation the next. Irritable bladder, or interstitial cystitis, causes frequent and sometimes painful urination. Gastroesophageal reflux disease (GERD) is also common among FM patients. And some sources state that about 50 percent of FM patients report heightened sensitivity to odors, noises, bright lights, medications, changes in the weather, and/or various foods. Finally, difficulty processing, understanding, and retaining information is another maddening and sometimes disabling symptom that many FM patients deal with every day. Whether this "fibro fog" is caused by stress, pain, sensory overload, fatigue, or our diet, we know there are times when we are unable to think straight or remember important facts.

Some people have fibromyalgia alone, but the illness can accompany other conditions such as chronic fatigue syndrome, rheumatoid arthritis, or osteoarthritis, among others.

Up to 25 percent of FM patients suffer from depression or anxiety. It isn't surprising that FM patients feel depressed. A chronic-pain condition changes your life. FM patients go through stages of grief after diagnosis (read more about this in Chapters 3 and 6). They may feel anxious about their treatment, their economic situation, the changes happening in their body. But FM is not a psychiatric disorder. Still, in the book *Fibromyalgia: The New Integrative Approach*, Milton Hammerly, M.D., tells us that "it is not uncommon to be told (or treated as if) 'it's all in your head.'" A familiar experience of people with FM is to hear the comment, "But how can you be sick? You look fine!" Fibromyalgia is an invisible illness, a fact that greatly contributes to the skepticism with which FM patients' very real symptoms are sometimes greeted by others—including family members, friends, coworkers, acquaintances, even medical professionals.

Hammerly continues, "Well, it's not in your head. In fact, it's all in your body—all *through* your body, potentially affecting many different systems, including your

◀ Musculoskeletal system

◀ Digestive system

◀ Immune system

◀ Circulatory system

◀ Endocrine system

◀ Nervous system

He further states, "To dismiss the far-reaching, multiple symptoms of fibromyalgia as being psychosomatic is not only insulting, it's potentially dangerous. A missed or incorrect diagnosis can lead to worsening symptoms and expose you to the unnecessary risks of improper treatment."

Fibromyalgia certainly is *not* a "wastebasket diagnosis." It exists; it's real; it's not "all in your head."

On the more positive side, fibromyalgia doesn't seem to be progressive, and it isn't contagious.

WHAT CAUSES FM?

Researchers and doctors disagree about the cause of FM. Some believe it is caused by a deficit in the neurotransmitter serotonin. Some believe it is a central-nervous-system dysfunction. (And, as alluded to above, others still don't believe it's a "real" illness.) Many studies are being conducted to learn more about the possible causes of FM, and new theories on the topic regularly appear in the news media.

FM may come on after a traffic accident or traumatic event. This is called *post-traumatic fibromyalgia*. Some women whose

stories appear in this book have described their symptoms as showing up after a life-changing event, such as divorce, surgery, or a
death in the family. By contrast, *primary FM* seems to come on
over time.

In my case, it all began with surgery on my feet, followed by a
severe case of giardiasis (from the intestinal parasite *Giardia*), and
an episode of chemical poisoning. I dropped a bottle of the pesticide Isotox, it shattered, and I cleaned it up. Over the next several
years I began to experience pain all over my body and fatigue that
wouldn't be relieved with sleep or rest.

Because individuals with FM usually are less active than they
once were, they can become deconditioned—or "out of shape"—
after the onset of FM, but it is important to remember that decon-
ditioning does not *cause* FM.

WHAT IS FM LIKE? SOME PERSPECTIVES

Here are a few women's perspectives on what it's like to live with
fibromyalgia, including an extended essay on the topic by Sisu G.:

Victoria M. The pain associated with FM is the most debilitating
aspect. It is frustrating. I cannot do the tasks I have always
enjoyed, such as gardening and housework; even shopping for
food is difficult. I am very creative in the home and garden—or at
least I was. I have always loved to do physical things, but after FM
I couldn't participate in sports, bushwalking, or anything that
required physical stamina. I have, however, pushed myself—particularly on the home front—and suffered the pain afterward, as I am
not one to sit back and watch life go by. Still, when I suffered from
CFS and FM together, there was no pushing myself. My body simply could not respond.

The benefits of having broadened my mind in earlier days—that
is, reading and learning about philosophy, mind behaviors, and
prayer—gave me mental strength, which supported me while my
body was so incredibly incapacitated.

Gerry L. I can tell you when it all began: at age forty-eight, during
menopause. The symptoms were bizarre. Ear noises, numbness,

tingling, burning pain in my face, weakness, "icy hot"—this is how I described what I was feeling. It is called a syndrome because of the myriad signs and symptoms that go with it, some so odd that we don't tell our doctors: IBS (irritable bowel syndrome), numbness/ tingling, weakness in arms or legs, depression, confusion, memory problems, trouble finding words, pelvic pain, pain during intimacy, restless legs, chills, flulike feelings, sensitivity to cold. It can be eighty degrees and I will be cold. You don't need a weather report. I will tell you when the humidity is increasing.

▲▲▲

Patricia's comments, below, include discussion of one of the most universally frustrating aspects of living with fibromyalgia: its invisibility. This is the characteristic of the illness that causes some doctors to tell those of us with FM that it's "all in our heads" and some family members to disbelieve that we are "really" sick.

Patricia S.   I am fifty two. I've had fibromyalgia all my life. I remember at a young age feeling some kind of pain and thinking, gee, does everybody feel like this? It just got worse as I got older. Now I'm really sick, and my muscles are in complete knots. I get a massage every week. My massage therapist says I'm in the worst shape of any client she's ever had. My muscles are like rocks, and yet at the same time my ligaments and tendons are too loose. I'm floppy all over the place and very loose, and my range of motion is good, but my muscles are ropes and rocks. That's what I think fibromyalgia is often about. It's that tension in the muscles, but you're unable to will them to relax. It's a chemical reaction in the muscle. I think a lot of the energy we've lost is stored in the muscles, keeping them contracted.

People do not understand my difficulties because I do not look sick. They ask me when I'm going back to work. They don't understand that I am not better. It is not like catching a cold and getting over it, nor is it like a chronic disease such as diabetes or heart disease that can often be well-managed and still allow you to work. There are no satisfactory treatments available for FM. Some days you feel like you can't get out of bed. Of course I do anyway, but I'm still not functioning at a high level. Since I do not work, most people think I am doing nothing and have all the world's time on my hands. They tell me to get involved with this or that project. It infuriates me that they fail to understand that taking care of myself and dealing with this syndrome is very time-consuming.

Sisu G. I never figured me for the kind to come down with an unknown mystery disease. I was the healthy girl, the one who'd taken a single sick day in three years, the one who the doctors weren't sure would walk after her spine injury but who did just fine. I was the girl so young and healthy that old people sighed on the subway. Fresh-faced, bright-eyed, with clear skin and energy to spare.

I'm not sure where that energy went. I feel pretty normal, most days, but once in a while I'll remember something I used to do, and it will contrast so vividly with what I can do now that it's a shock.

Would you believe that it all started with a cough? Really. This whole mess started with a light cough that wouldn't go away but wasn't bad enough to bother me. I was working two retail jobs at the time; how's that for energy? And I was cheerful, I was helpful, and I did my work well. I came down with a cough in the spring two years ago and thought nothing of it till the next October, when I came down with a real cold. The cough happened only once in a while; it was a light cough, a catch in my throat; I couldn't quite get my breath properly. But then I caught cold and got a nasty chest cough and a fever. I tried to keep working. I'd changed jobs by then. I just couldn't do retail. I was more and more tired, and it was getting harder and harder to catch my breath. So I switched to office work. But I got this cold and this fever, and my friends put me to bed, and when I got better I still had this cough, only now it was serious and my chest hurt.

I didn't have a doctor. When you're healthy for so long and have no health insurance, who needs a doctor? I didn't even know how to go to a doctor. Or where to find one. So I didn't. And I would wake up at night coughing, gasping, feeling no air in my lungs.

My best friend finally took me to the emergency room. I thought I might die. They thought I might die, too, and strapped me to a stretcher while they tried to figure out what was wrong. My breathing normalized. They did asthma tests. No asthma. They gave me inhalers anyway. After that I couldn't stay healthy. Every week it was a cold, a flu virus, something. I got head colds that lasted months. They ran HIV/AIDS tests that turned up negative. I was too tired to function. I'd get home from work and collapse. No one understood what was happening to me.

And then we got to talking about my hands. See, my hands have hurt for years. And my feet have hurt when I wake up in the morning for so many years that I thought it was normal. I would wake up and put my feet to the ground and they'd hurt so badly. When I was eighteen, I read the story of the Little Mermaid, where she's told that walking on the mortal earth will cut her like knives. And that startled me; I knew how that felt. I'm not supposed to know what that's like, am I? That was my first inkling that this problem with my feet wasn't normal, but it didn't resurface in my mind till the doctors and I got to talking about how tired I was and how my hands hurt.

Then my hands started shaking. I thought maybe it was the inhalers. My hands would occasionally twitch; I'd drop things. God, I thought, am I coming down with something really awful? When I worked on my car, my hands shook so badly that I cried. Yet still I felt "normal." It's amazing how normal you feel, even when drastic, real things are happening to you. The sense of self is very elastic. So I finally went in and made the doctor take notes on all of this. By this point I had doctors, all right. They don't let you out of the emergency room without follow-up when you go in with breathing problems. I'd even switched to a different medical center when it didn't look like the first one had a clue. They started doing blood tests.

In six months I'd given up everything from makeup to perfume in the attempt to be able to breathe. There were times when I was too tired to move. And random, sharp pains. And my hands.... Something was happening, and no one could tell me what. But then my sister was diagnosed with celiac disease—a chronic nutritional disorder characterized by an intolerance to gluten—so I got tested for it too. I tested positive. Finally I had an explanation for why my immune system had been going crazy for more than a year. And for all the allergies and chemical sensitivities I'd developed. Now maybe people would think I was a sci-fi freak, a biologically bizarre specimen, with all my sensitivities and allergies and intolerances, but at least it was something specific. Life could return to normal.

My breathing got better, but my hands didn't. In fact, they got worse. My hands and feet had been getting worse all along, and by the time the celiac diagnosis came in, they were going numb. I had worked as an office temp all through this. What do you do when you're twenty-five, have never been to college, have been spending all your income on medications and doctors, and your sole means of work is your typing and office skills? I had to carry things carefully so as not to drop them. I remember trying to file, trying to look nonchalant as I swallowed my rising fear about my frozen hands. I could move them, but it was like typing with gloves on. And your balance suffers when you can't feel the floor evenly. It was a difficult time.

Fortunately, I had good doctors. When a young woman can't feel her fingers, the doctors worry, because it usually means something bad. So they started more testing. They tested for lupus; they tested for MS. I felt as numb inwardly as my hands did outwardly. How could I have MS? Or lupus? How could I have any of the nasty things those tests look for? I'm so young. So healthy. But so tired. The doctors hated it, too. Seeing a girl who looks healthy and alive and yet has something drastically wrong with her demonstrates a fundamental fracture in the way things are supposed to be. The doctor who performed the electromyograms on me hated to do it, hated to jab me with the needles, hated to send the current through my limbs. But we had to; there was no other way. Those were the painful tests. They hurt a lot, and they are frightening. You know they wouldn't be testing your nerves if they didn't think something might be wrong with them. By this point I was so tired that I couldn't do anything but work, and I was hard-pressed to make it through my days. I would come home and collapse. I couldn't walk four blocks, and I was so tired I sometimes couldn't make it up the stairs. I promised myself I'd stop working if I got so tired that I couldn't brush my teeth.

The next night, I couldn't brush my teeth. I kept working and bought an electric toothbrush.

But there was another piece to this that had seemed normal at the time: sleep. The twitches I always had at night that woke me up? Those aren't normal either, it turns out. They used to happen once or twice a night, every night. Over the last five years it had gotten worse, and I hadn't paid attention. But one day my doctor and I talked about my sleep patterns. And that was when I realized that it had been three years since I'd had anything like halfway decent sleep. Probably five or six years since I'd had a somewhat regular sleep pattern. I was stunned. I'd gone two years without a decent night's sleep? In fact, it had been more than a year since I'd gotten even five hours of deep sleep a night.

The pieces fell together as all the tests—the blood tests, the scans, the screenings—came in and were handed to my new doctor, a rheumatologist. At this point the numbness was starting to be replaced by pain, and I was getting desperate. I prayed that I didn't have MS or lupus.

My strange collection of symptoms turned out to be fibromyalgia, a mysterious chronic-pain syndrome. And it isn't degenerative, but I'd been getting steadily worse for months, and the rheumatologist was very open about the fact that I might continue to do so. He also told me there are doctors who don't believe this is a real illness.

Great. Not only do I get an incurable disease, but I get one nobody believes in. Not only does no one understand how it happens or why, but there is no cure because some doctors aren't even looking.

I did get worse, for six or seven months, and then we managed to slow it down and stop it. Stop what? Well, that's the thing. No one's quite sure. There are a lot of models proposed about how FM might work. It might be circulatory, with the chemicals that are built up by movement never getting cleared away, since FM patients don't get the fourth-stage sleep that lets the growth hormones for healing get secreted. Or it might be neurochemical—my body creates three to four times the pain chemicals of a normal person; we know that much. It might be an infection—from a virus, from bacteria, or even from a mycoplasma (a group of parasitic microorganisms that in some respects are intermediate between viruses and bacteria). As science has found new ways to examine the symptoms, more attention is being paid to the reality of FM.

This illness was unheard of in the past. That's different now. Changes in reporting procedures, changes in diagnostic criteria, and changes in technology that allow for evidence of a whole new kind to be presented have all altered the medical landscape. Fibromyalgia is just one of the murky pools that has become a solid mountain range in the process. Now there is so much to find out that no one knows where to start.

That said, what is it like?

It hurts. It opens up a whole new realm of pain. This isn't like a headache or a broken arm. It isn't something solid, like a broken foot. It is like I just ran five miles and topped it off with a bout of weightlifting. Right now I'm tired, I'm sore, and I feel like I have the flu. But with FM I always feel like that; this is nothing new. Yet it's unlike having the flu, because I don't just sleep it off or feel weird for a day. And you can't push through it, because that makes it worse. It's a lot like having bad arthritis. My hands hurt a lot, and I get pretty stiff sometimes. It can hurt to do things. Yet sometimes I feel almost fine. It rises and falls; it ends up feeling pretty normal. It doesn't affect who I am—that's the weird thing. I'm still in here.

Here's what a typical day with FM is like for me. I usually wake up at six. I set my clothes out the night before, so I won't have to think first thing in the morning and also because there's no extra energy for ironing in the morning. I take my shower the night before. Without the Flexeril (a prescription muscle relaxant), it really hurts to get out of bed. It's the worst when my feet hit the floor—I experience a sharp pain, like the soles of my feet have worn through. And I feel stiff and awkward. My joints and muscles hurt. But without the Flexeril the pain is a lot worse. I also awaken feeling awfully foggy.

The first place I go is to the kitchen to put water on for tea. Then I get dressed. I don't usually wear makeup anymore; I gave that up without thinking about it, because I haven't had the necessary energy in a long time. Getting breakfast—which consists of something instant (there's no way I could cook)—and getting myself out the door are serious tasks, especially with my mental acuity so blunted in the morning. I've made my lunch the night before. Got my badge, got my keys, got my lunch, got my tai chi clothes (if it's Tuesday or Thursday). My bus pass is attached to my keys. I leave and catch the bus.

I work forty hours a week. I'm a rare one. Most people with this illness aren't so lucky. But I have a good job: I can sit down and rest, and there's very little mental or emotional stress. It isn't challenging. I like that; I have enough challenge just keeping my life together. It hurts my arms and shoulders to type; it's a wearing pain, a dull one, on the best days. (We'll talk about the bad days later. Right now I have mostly good days.) I leave work at four. I take the train to tai chi (two stops) or home. When I get home, I rest for half an hour before trying to cook dinner. I'm too tired and in too much pain for the first fifteen minutes to even think.

That's the other part: the fog. Pain brings on a mental density of its own, but beyond that there's a cognitive difficulty that goes with this illness. It's a lot like waking up and not having any coffee. You stare at the coffeepot for five minutes trying to remember what you're supposed to do with it. You wander down the grocery aisle trying to remember what you're there for. Oh, everybody does that, I know. But I do it every day. Crossword puzzles are a bitch; I lose nouns when I'm tired or in pain. My roomie laughs and says if we had a dollar for every time I asked for that...that...that...thing, there, or the thing, you know, that you use for...—followed by a pantomime act. It isn't so bad in the morning, after I've been up for a couple of hours and before I'm exhausted.

Before I go to bed, I have to get my clothes out for the next day and make my lunch. These things take a while when you have to go slowly and remember what you're doing. My arms get to feeling rubbery by that point in the day, and I start to ache all over. I have to really pay attention, because that's the edge, right there. I've found out the hard way that if I do too much, there's another kind of pain. There's the ache, and there's the tingling kind of pain, and then there's a whole different kind—the kind that feels like spikes. Sudden, fierce stabs in random places. One in my hand. As it begins to fade, I feel one in my foot. Or my shoulder. Or my ribs. Or maybe a knee, or my other wrist. And then another. And another. They are like muscle cramps without the twitch, like a charley horse without the cramping, like a railroad spike through the flesh. But there's nothing there. This illness is full of phantom attacks, pain that feels like events. The pains will eventually subside; they won't get fainter but they'll get farther apart. I lie real still and let it pass—the more I can relax my muscles, the less I'll contribute to the pain. That's one of the prices for overdoing things. It hurts more than anything. It feels real, and once it starts, it takes a while to stop. My painkillers don't touch it. I haven't tried the new pill on it yet, but I'm being careful so I don't have to.

Then there are the bad days. On a bad day, during a flare, everything hurts. I have an inflammation in my rib cage sometimes, called costochondritis. It's not fatal. Ibuprofen sometimes helps with it. Feels like a cracked rib. In fact, doctors do a lot of X rays to rule out a cracked rib when they diagnose it. On a bad day I don't count the kinds of pain. Things just hurt. I feel old. I shouldn't feel this way at my age. My doctors and nurses all have great compassion; they don't play "poor you" at me, but they know I've lost a lot of the fun I should be having, and gained a lot of issues I shouldn't be facing till I'm sixty—if I weren't taking care of myself then, that is.

Flares feel just like they sound. Like solar flares. Storms. Pain storms. Things just aren't calm—there's one thing and another, and you take your meds and hope for the best and try to take it easy. They are strings of bad days, held together by the wish to just lie down and rest and feel better, by the attempt to remember what it felt like to look down a street and not have to decide whether to walk. To know that you once could get up and dance to a song without worrying that you wouldn't be able to cook dinner.

You get a limited energy budget with this illness. You can spend it any way you want, but if you overspend, there's hell to pay. Sometimes there's hell to pay anyway. The things that can cause a flare are legion. And sometimes they're anonymous—you wake up and your carefully kept health balance has tipped. But a sure thing that will bring on a flare is cold weather or wet weather. Heat is my friend; I frequently feel cold, and it's awful. I feel as if my skeleton were frozen; I can never get warm enough. Immersion in water below eighty-eight degrees can cause a flare. So can lifting heavy objects. Walking too far at one time. Walking too far, period. Emotional stress. Did I mention that my body no longer handles stress? The chemicals involved in stress reactions are very much like the ones involved in overexertion, I guess. Stress produces those knifelike, horrible pains. A long cry can start a flare. A crying bout is something I pay for by sitting still while the pains come and go until they are done. I have to try not to get into bad moods.

The good stuff can result in overexertion, too. I'm to avoid shocks. Even parties can exhaust me. A dinner party gets calculated—the higher the number of guests, the shorter the time I can stay. Meetings at work get deducted from my energy budget. So

does grocery shopping. I have to plan my week carefully. Laundry is something I do on a day when I don't plan to do anything else.
 And that's what it's like.

▲▲▲

Okay, you may be thinking, but where's the *good* news? What can I *do* about all this? In fact, there is much a person can do to alleviate the symptoms of FM. Keep reading; later chapters in the book address those very issues. For now, let's meet other women who tell us their stories in these pages.

CHAPTER

2

A Community of Women

To prepare for this book I made a list of women I knew who were living with fibromyalgia. Some were acquaintances, one was a friend, another was a family member, and several were women who had written to me after reading *Alternative Treatments for Fibromyalgia and Chronic Fatigue Syndrome*. It was a short list, so to find more potential participants I asked the wonderful folks at www.ImmuneSupport.com (sponsored by Pro Health, Inc.; see Resources) to place a notice in their online magazine. Suddenly more women were responding than I knew what to do with!

Altogether, fifty-three women answered the survey I'd prepared. (A copy of the survey appears at the end of this chapter.) Most responded by e-mail, but some wrote letters in longhand. A couple of women said they found it therapeutic to complete the questionnaire; doing so caused them to look at the changes brought about by their illness in a more complete way. Two women responded a little bit each night for a week. I looked forward to each posting, which revealed these women answer by answer.

The correspondence represented people at many different points on the spectrum of illness and recovery. One woman sent a short e-mail message that began with her name and city. Her only words after that were "Please help me." I answered by suggesting every possible way I could think of to help her, but I never heard back from her.

THE WOMEN

Below are brief bios of the thirty-eight women whose stories appear in these pages. Some of the women used their real names, and some preferred to use pseudonyms. It is my hope that their words in the context of this book offer help and hope. However, as is consistently exemplified in the testimonies of these women living with fibromyalgia, you must take the first step.

▲▲▲

Alison H. I live in Lexington, Kentucky. I attend the University of Kentucky full-time as a social-work major. I work part-time. I am twenty years old and single.

The most positive emotion I have felt since my diagnosis with FM is being able to relate to someone else. Knowing that I am not alone is the best therapy. I have also had to get to know myself better so as to deal with all of the things going on in my body. I have had to really evaluate what I put my trust in and what I devote my time to, and it has led to some amazing self-discovery.

Every day, my motivation to keep going comes from the fact that there are tons of people out there whom I can help. Tons of people who are worse off than me. Tons of people who can help me as well. There is still so much to learn, and I know God has a plan for my life, so I just have to trust that. My reward comes from conquering a desire to give in and give up. My reward comes from helping others and not focusing on myself. My reward comes when I can feel good about my decisions and not overwork my body. And my reward comes from knowing that I have persevered.

Carol J. I live in Red Oak, Iowa. I am fifty-six. I was a hairstylist for thirty-three years. FM certainly slowed my business. I worked through such pain and fatigue it is a wonder I didn't really screw up someone's hair! Over the years my work hours shortened and eventually I had to withdraw completely from working. Today I maintain a website for people with fibromyalgia.

Charlene M. I live in Loveland, Ohio, with my mother and my son. I have two children and three grandchildren. I am involved in my church and attend Bible-study groups, which have become a good part of my support system.

Cheryl R. I am forty-four and live in Melbourne, Florida, with my husband of fifteen years, Ron, and our two cats, CD and Kattie Lynn. Our home is about ten minutes from the ocean, and we love living here. I was forced to quit my job as a self-employed glass etcher. In addition to my health problems, my husband needs a liver transplant.

I pray for everyone who must live with FM. Especially if one lacks a team of good and knowledgeable doctors, this illness is nearly impossible to deal with. I find life calm right now due to the confidence I have in our own health-care team and, of course, thanks to a whole lot of prayer.

Cheryl W. I am a former tennis professional from Florida; my undergraduate work was in physical education. I became interested in myotherapy when a sports injury kept me from playing tennis. After exploring alternative therapies, including surgery, I found that myotherapy was the only treatment that alleviated the pain and enabled me to resume a pain-free, physically active life. I am a certified trigger-point therapist and exercise therapist.

Cybill C. I live in Vinland, New Jersey, and am divorced with three kids. I am a registered nurse. My life has changed drastically since FM. Before, I was full of energy. I worked three jobs and had an active social life, as well as being a wife and mother. Now I've had to cut so many activities from my life that I feel as though I am at the mercy of FM.

Cydney B. I am fifty-four. I am married with two daughters and live in Algona, Iowa. I was diagnosed in 1994. I was a human-resources manager for my whole career, after getting a bachelor's degree in psychology. I moved up, albeit more slowly than most non-child-laden women, and ended up as a senior manager/lower-level director at a large, famous biotech company. I had my dream job. I'd been in it for two and a half years. I had made it. Then, wham, rheumatoid arthritis and fibromyalgia hit—and no job. I remember thinking on my way to work once before I got sick, "Life is going too well. Something awful is going to happen." Thoughts of an orphan child, I guess.

Denise P. I am fifty-three years old and live in Fort Bragg, California. I work for the county social-services department, administering grant programs such as cash aid, food stamps, and medical services. I am single with one daughter and a grandson.

My tip for readers is to try not to let FM get you down. Do as much as you can, and just keep going. Find something you can do to help take your mind off the pain and other symptoms. I stay as active as possible in my community grange. I go to meetings and serve as secretary. We host a breakfast on the first Sunday of each month, and I try to attend and to help in any way I can.

Diane H. I am fifty-five and a former assistant attorney general. I live in southern Arizona with my husband, who is retired. I miss being able to play golf and go hiking, but I enjoy reading, writing, walking, and volunteering my legal services.

Since participating in a scientific study sponsored by the University of Arizona College of Medicine to research whether homeopathic remedies help fibromyalgia, I'm sleeping better and feeling better than I have in years. I'm unable to work; I mostly choose to enjoy my husband's retirement while he's still healthy. I've found that attitude is everything, and I'm doing fine.

Learn to let go. If you can't get it done, let it go. If you can't do it all, let it go. When you feel better, do less.

Donna F. I am a thirty-six-year-old wife and mother of four. I've learned that no matter what your circumstance, no matter what your amount of suffering, the human spirit is more driven than I was previously aware. I've learned there is hope even when you think it can't get any worse. I've learned as a woman that more than perfect health keeps me going—I'm also motivated by my family and my drive to achieve goals and to keep up with life because it includes me and I want to enjoy it.

Donna P. I live in Richland, Washington. I am single and live with my two cats. I also have two sons. I was in law enforcement for a good part of my earlier life. After I became sick, I decided to go into retail. I had a poor attendance record, but I did not get fired. I always had a doctor's slip to prove I was ill. I worked in linens at a large department store, and I loved every minute of it. I liked to work with people and help them with their purchases. Now every time I go to that department store, I cry. I loved working.

I hope to learn more about the computer and maybe write a book someday. Life is slower for me now. I take time to enjoy the day, watch the birds, see the beautiful sunsets, and just look at the world with a different attitude. One way to look at being disabled is to appreciate the fact that you have lots of free time. When I have good days, I really enjoy not having to get up and hurry to get ready.

Donna S. I am the primary caretaker for my husband, Don, who has fibromyalgia. We live in a small town in Ohio and have two children. I appreciate the fact that, when his health permits it, Don can stay home and take care of our son and the house. I have spent years researching Don's condition.

Donnie M. I live in Wilmington, North Carolina, with my husband. Acceptance is the main thing I have had to learn in order to cope. I am fortunate to have a husband who is supportive and helps me with so many things. I could not manage without him. My love and appreciation for my husband has grown.

Emma L. I live in Mountain View, California, and am sixty-five years old. I was born and grew up in Italy. I came to the U.S. in 1960. I have been a business manager since 1973. I am bilingual and am a translator of English into Italian and vice versa. I also speak French and Spanish. I married a Hungarian man, my second husband, in 1991.

I am not American by culture or training. My attitude about life, problems, health, and everything else is not the same as that prevalent in this country.

Just as I never was a person who embraced ritual or routine, I also never had long-term plans or goals. There were always things I desired to do, and I figured out how to do them, but mostly I responded to circumstances as they happened and solved problems as they arose. In a real way, this prepared me well for the demands of FM. My main problem now is that I cannot figure out how I could possibly live in France, which is what I would really like to do. Unfortunately, I am not even strong enough to go to the corner store!

Gerry L. I am fifty-eight and live in Lemont, Illinois, a suburb of Chicago. I have been married for thirty-seven years to my high school sweetheart. We have a daughter and a son. Nursing was my passion. I worked in hospitals, all shifts. I worked in same-day surgery and as a home-health case manager. I touched lives and made a difference. And I learned from my patients things you don't learn in books. I have quotes from them and their families. I attended many wakes and held hands so no one died alone. I was such a good nurse. I wasn't through yet, but it was taken from me. Why? I don't know. Because. There is no answer to the question why. But every once in a while, I think maybe it's because I am supposed to help others in ways different from nursing. I continue to grieve my loss.

Pain is my companion but it is not me. I must make choices. I may not enjoy each day as much as I used to, but I sure try to embrace each one. I can't be miserable all of the time.

Gina H. I am forty-eight years old and have two sons. I reside in Columbus, Georgia, and I have been married for twenty-one years.

I am currently not working because of my fibromyalgia. After almost twelve years as a school crossing guard, I had to resign because I could no longer raise my left arm. I needed both hands and arms to direct traffic and help children cross. I loved my job. I directed anywhere from 250 to 300 cars and crossed about 100 kids every day. But with the pain of FM I just could not do it any more. That hurt me badly because I really enjoyed being in control out there.

Ginger C. I live in Olney, Illinois. I am forty-one and have three children. I have had to slow down a lot. I don't have the energy I did before, but I find that a positive attitude helps me. I am determined that I will not let this disease beat me. Either I can learn to live with it, or it can control me, and I won't let that happen.

Jean T. I live in Spokane, Washington. I turned seventy years old (how did that happen?) in April 2002. Even with my illness, I don't feel old in my mind and heart. I am retired (under protest) only because I simply don't have the stamina I used to have. I am an interior designer and I have my real estate broker's license.

When my husband was very ill just before he passed away, he was sort of talking to himself when he said, "I had so many things I wanted to do and places I wanted to go. I guess I will do them in the next world." I don't think he knew I was in the room. It does make me take note of the important things I still want to do. Yet I am not scared. I have done a lot of research and I don't feel I have anything to fear.

Katie G. I live in Kirkland, Washington, and am single. My lifestyle has changed a lot. Since my illness/diagnosis, I have learned how very strong I truly am. I am a survivor—for the long haul. I have incredible endurance, self-reliance, perseverance, and determination. My drive and will get me through a lot and keep me focused forward. I can amuse myself, laugh with and at myself. The skills and experiences I've gained through this illness will be invaluable throughout the remainder of my life.

It is my current job and responsibility to rise above this illness that mystifies the medical community and to make life better for myself. I realize that although I feel my full potential isn't being fulfilled, other parts of myself are being developed that wouldn't necessarily be if I hadn't gotten fibromyalgia and chronic fatigue syndrome.

Kay B. I live in Janesville, Wisconsin, with my husband, Tim. Am I happy with my life as it is? No. Am I thankful? Yes. I love my husband and my family, and the people who matter are around me. I have learned to take joy in the faces of my family when I cook supper for them, and they enjoy the food that is sometimes hard for me to make. I have my life, which is fulfilling. I have lots more time to pray. I work hard every day at the computer, trying to reeducate my brain so I can do the thinking I once was able to do. I find great satisfaction in the fact that I am relearning to learn.

I pray more. I talk to God more. I am quietly peaceful in my heart for the first time in my life. Would I be here in my head and heart if I were not ill? I don't think so. I have learned to live that sappy poem they use in twelve-step programs: I have gained the ability to live a day at a time and to be thankful for that day. The future will come a day at a time whether I think about it or not!

Lalenya R. I live in Heathrow, Florida. Before my disease I was a marketing director, and I traveled throughout the state. I worked out four times a week and was in great shape for a fifty-year-old woman. After being single for many years, I met a wonderful man whom I married in 1997. In 1998, my doctor placed me on disability and my life changed substantially. I am no longer able to work out, which used to provide a great endorphin high. My social interactions have been curtailed greatly, and I find myself becoming more isolated. I have never been one to dwell on health issues or complain of the constant pain, so it's easier to be alone than with people who can't understand the disease.

Linda M. I am a former trade-magazine columnist and author of two best-selling cookbooks. I was in a car accident in 1987. The collision triggered fibromyalgia. The pain of FM has driven some people to suicide. I found myself writing poetry instead. In 1996, I published *Poetry of Pain,* a unique health/inspirational book for pain sufferers, caretakers, health professionals, and people who care.

In 1995, I was part of the Washington State Department of Health committee to write new state guidelines for chronic-pain management. I am a board member of the Washington Intractable Chronic Pain Association. I am married to a fisherman and have two sons.

Lindamarie M. I live in Brighton, Maine, with my husband and daughter. I have been living with FM for over thirteen years. I am thirty-nine years old.

Marcia D. I am fifty-one and married to Joe, with a son, Stacy, and a daughter, Jamie. We live in Milwaukie, Oregon, and Heppner, Oregon.

It's my stubbornness that keeps me going. I stay as independent as I can. I strive to keep an open mind about all of this; I'll try anything new to see if it will help. A lot of days I get really depressed, but I try to take one day at a time. Some days are better than others.

Mary H.-B. I am a wife, a mother, and a program analyst for the federal government. I am thirty-seven and live in Sunderland, Maryland. I have started a support group. I spend time each day doing research to help others get more control of their lives with FM/CFS. I have a loving husband and four beautiful children to remind me that life is very short.

Mea C. I am thirty-five years old, married to a wonderful man, and the mother of a teenage son. We live in Wisconsin, a beautiful state. I wouldn't want to live anywhere else.

I started having symptoms when I was twenty-three, and they continued to get worse. Six years ago I went from doctor to doctor, but none of them could tell me what was wrong. One doctor made me so angry by telling me my pain was all in my head that I ended up kicking him in the shin. Not a good thing in hindsight, but it helped me at the time!

Nancy D. I have one son and live in Belfair, Washington. What drives me forward is that things have to be done; I live for others, who live for me. I wish to create fun projects outdoors, and I hope to have more visitors to my home. I was lucky to find a piece of property that offers serenity and a chance to create. I also go forward with hope that I can find a partner and with hope that I will see my family sometime. It is somehow held together by the miracles I have seen happen—I know they are there. I hope to learn more than I know now. Knowledge is always worth the effort. The reward in my life is that I have a great son. I also have my parents, who have proven their love for me in many ways. My comfortable home is another reward.

Norah T. I live in Mountlake Terrace, Washington, and have three grown children. I am a psychotherapist. From the outset, I inform my clients that I am disabled by fibromyalgia, migraines, and a metabolic disorder. The most essential service I offer to my clients is validation that their fibromyalgia is real and that something can and should be done about their pain and fatigue. During those times when I feel limited by my health, it helps me to know that I can give to someone else.

Patricia S. I am fifty-two years old and from Florida. I am single. Prior to becoming disabled I was an anesthesiologist. I was diagnosed with FM in 1985. I am also dealing with vulvodynia, which is severe vaginal pain.

I have learned that I am more of an optimist than I thought I was. I can't and won't give up hope. I never thought like that before.

Penny G. I am fifty-one and work as a waitress and sales associate. I am married to Chuck and have three children, Brian (twenty-six), Michael (twenty-three), and Sarah (eleven). I went back to school and received an associate degree in marketing with a 4.0 GPA five days after my fiftieth birthday.

I am a Christian and I believe God wants me to enjoy what I can. I am visually moved as an artist and I also enjoy writing. I am working on my own story and seek to publish it when it is finished.

I know that I will be able to do less and less, and if that is the answer, I will find the courage to be my best self in spite of my health problems. If I can no longer draw, I will take photos. If I can no longer act, I will attend plays. If I can no longer work, I will volunteer. I will always enjoy our beautiful world; if I can't take leisurely walks, I will sit on a park bench. God bless.

Rachel B. I am thirty-one years old and am an occupational-therapy manager. I am married. We live in Pratt, Kansas. My partner and I have been together for five years; for two of those I've had FM. I'm glad my partner knew the person I was before FM, and at times I get reminders that I'm not that person anymore. I do not know if I ever will be that person again.

My doctor also suspects that I have multiple sclerosis. When one flares up, so does the other. Separately, their symptoms seem moderate. Together, they are severe and hard to control. This makes it very challenging for the doctor and a rough road for me.

I am an RN, a mental-health therapist, an energy practitioner, and a writer. I live in Port Orchard, Washington, with my husband and cats. I am fifty three years old.

I maintain a part-time job and am putting in what amounts to almost full-time hours on my book project, in addition to doing the bulk of managing the home. My life remains very busy. I take time out for myself in the following ways: treadmill walking, long "prayer-time" showers that include energy work, journaling, reading, and prayer in the evening.

Sisu G. I am twenty-five years old. I work as a security reception-ist. I am single. I live just outside of Boston, Massachusetts.

I usually spend at least an hour a day reading up on this illness and all the studies being done, and I post some of that info where my friends can see it, to help them better understand.

Sondra H. I live in Arlington, Texas. I am thirty-seven years old and was diagnosed with FM four years ago. I work as an executive producer in broadcast television. I have two teenage daughters and a very understanding husband. I went through a four-month program for sufferers of chronic pain at the University of Texas Southwest Medical Center. What they taught me has been invalu-able to my well-being and has made me cope with the condition and continue on the path of managing my health, family, and work.

Dealing with FM on a daily basis becomes a lifestyle. At first it's difficult because you are rethinking and reevaluating everything you do. After time, as with any training, it becomes second nature. Granted, there are still times when you stumble, but you pick your-self up and get back on track. Important things to me include knowing how to deal with stress and listening to my body. I use meditation to relax. Taking small amounts of time throughout the day to regroup and relax helps.

I treat each day as a blessing; doing so motivates me. Seeing my family and friends and enjoying the small things we often over-look—those are my rewards. How often do people take time to marvel at the way a hawk soars, or how the light bounces off blades of grass, or the way your kids confide in you? Maybe it's the way the dogs welcome you and love you—they never have a bad day, even if you do. Life offers so many rewards. FM just helped me to see them and appreciate them a little more. I think I enjoyed these same things before FM, but nowhere to the degree I do now. My essence and spirit have been impacted by FM. I've been able to sift through many layers of myself, and I wouldn't trade who I am now for anything.

Sonia H. I am sixty-nine years old, and I live in Kirkland, Washington. I do editing and proofreading as a freelance independent contractor. Before FM, I was in real estate and I owned a flower shop. I became ill in 1989. At the time, I was working very long hours at my flower shop and taking care of an ailing parent, and I just collapsed after a particularly busy period and ended up in the hospital.

Generally, my friends are very supportive of me. I don't know that they totally understand the FM, but they believe me when I say I am too tired to go to the movies—although it has taken a while to get to that point. I think in the beginning they just couldn't imagine why I couldn't do what I used to do, but now they are very accepting of it.

Suzan B. I am forty-one and I live in Seattle, Washington, with my cat named Rabbit. Before fibromyalgia and CFIDS (chronic fatigue and immune dysfunction syndrome), I was an auto mechanic, a microbiologist at a biotech company, and a white-water raft guide. I have found spirituality to be the most important means of ensuring my survival. It is important to me to know I can be happy no matter what is happening on a physical plane.

Val T. I am a mother of two and a grandmother. I was diagnosed with FM in 1998, after a severe automobile accident. I am also dealing with hypothyroidism. I am a nurse working part-time in a medical clinic. I take care of patients of all ages who have varying degrees of illness. I'm on my feet running from the time I get there till the time I leave. I have also been giving speeches endorsing the success of my current pain treatment.

Victoria M. I am forty-six and the mother of two—Mathew, twenty, and Sarah, seventeen. I have been married to my husband, David, for almost twenty-four years. I live in Perth, Australia, capital of the territory of Western Australia and the most isolated capital city in the world. I have been here almost ten years, having moved across the country to live in a sunny climate by the seaside without much hustle or bustle.

By virtue of necessity, I slowed down the speed of my life. I haven't worked for five years. I do not make plans, as it disappoints me if I let myself or someone else down. I have a gorgeous dog who loves me unconditionally, has spent her whole life sleeping with me, and knows all my sadness and joys. My children's health is precarious, so I became a survivor determined to beat whatever we had in order to raise them and see them into adulthood. I hung on because of my beautiful children. I had to be there for them.

Wendy K. I work as a supervisor in the civilian division of a law-enforcement agency. I love working in the yard and planting flowers, and I draw much joy from my cat and dog.

THE SURVEY

Here is the questionnaire the women responded to. As Devin Starlanyl suggests in the Foreword, you might consider writing down the answers to these questions for yourself. Doing so may offer you some new perspectives on living with fibromyalgia. At the very least, it may prove therapeutically cathartic.

1. How did you feel when you were first told you had FM?

2. What has changed in your life since your FM diagnosis, as compared to before you were ill? How has your lifestyle changed since your diagnosis?

3. How long do you think you had FM before you were diagnosed?

4. Approximately seven out of every ten FM patients are women. Do you have any ideas about why this is the case?

5. How does FM impact your menstrual cycle? How has it affected menopause for you, if applicable?

6. Do you have any other illnesses or conditions in addition to FM? If so, how do they interact with FM?

7. What kinds of treatments, medications, or therapies are you currently receiving? How many have you tried and given up on?

8. How much time is dedicated to taking care of yourself? Give us an example of a typical day.

9. What are your coping strategies for dealing with FM? Give us a few tips for the newly diagnosed patient. What works for pain? For fatigue?

10. Are you able to take care of yourself independently? If not, who is helping you? Do you have a husband or partner?

11. What have you learned about yourself as a woman since your diagnosis?

12. Do you feel you are coping with FM differently from how a man would?

13. Discuss the feelings that have been most impacted (positively or negatively) by FM.

14. Have you identified your particular life stressors and are you actively dealing with them?

15. Talk about your emotions. Are you mad? Are you scared? Do you feel alone? What do you resent most? What other emotions are impacted by having FM?

16. Tell us about the everyday things you do that help and make a real difference in dealing with FM.

17. Tell us the creative things you do to make yourself feel better (e.g., arts, crafts, dancing, etc.).

18. Describes FM's impact on your relationships with your partners, children, extended family, friends.

19. As a woman with FM, has your role in the family changed?

20. Whom do you rely on most for your primary care? What is your relationship like with this care provider? Does the fact that you are a woman have an impact on this relationship or on the care you receive? Is this person a medical doctor?

21. Do you have a support network? What is it like? Who are the key people in your support network?

22. Do you feel understood and accepted?

23. Do you feel your illness is the result of a specific trauma or event? If so, please describe it.

24. When were you diagnosed, and what made you see a doctor?

25. How did you find this care provider?

26. Do you trust your care provider? Why or why not?

27. Do you feel societal pressures as a result of your FM diagnosis? As a woman with FM?

28. Tell us about your job/career and the impact FM has had on it.

29. If you are still working, do your coworkers know about your illness? How has FM changed your workplace relationships? Has your employer provided any accommodations? Do you feel you are still making positive contributions at your place of work?

30. What financial challenges have you faced as a result of having FM?

31. Are you receiving financial assistance? If so, which of the following do you receive: state-sponsored funds, social security disability, SSI benefits, or private/employer-provided insurance? Have you had to take any form of legal action to gain benefits? Was it hard to admit that you needed the help?

32. Compare the goals you had before your illness with the ones you have established since diagnosis.

33. Tell us about any positive emotional experiences you have had since your FM diagnosis.

34. How has FM affected you on a spiritual level? What thoughts do you have about the future?

35. Now that you have FM, what tips do you have for dealing with the normal, daily challenges of life?

36. What do you do for yourself beyond treating your FM? What drives you forward every day? What are your rewards in life?

The Relief of a Diagnosis

In response to the question asking what symptoms made them see a doctor in the beginning, all the women who answered my survey listed the following in some combination: allover body pain, fatigue, difficulty falling asleep and/or staying asleep, memory problems, and loss of ability to think straight. They wanted to know if these symptoms could be related.

So many women have spent so many years unsuccessfully chasing the pain and symptoms of fibromyalgia with inaccurate, ineffective, and sometimes condescending medical advice that when they finally are diagnosed with FM, one of their primary emotions is relief: "I'm so relieved there's a name attached to what I'm experiencing" or "I'm so relieved someone finally hears what I'm saying" or even "I knew I wasn't crazy."

But the relief of a diagnosis is just the beginning. For many women, myself included, fast on the heels of this reaction follow others: fear, anger, shock, loss. And then come the initial steps of learning to live with FM. This chapter addresses all these issues and more.

REACHING A DIAGNOSIS

My diagnosis came by way of a chance meeting with a podiatrist. In 1988, I began to experience strange foot pain. The pain started in one foot, but soon both of my feet hurt constantly. It was a burning, tingling, swollen, stabbing pain that increased the more I stood, and especially if I stood in one place for more than a few minutes—a real problem since I worked as a florist. Early on I was told I had sprained my foot, or that I had gout, or maybe a stress fracture. Eventually I was diagnosed with tarsal tunnel syndrome.

After several years of unrelenting discomfort, surgery seemed an option to consider. Back then, surgery for tarsal tunnel syndrome was considered by many to be a "cure," but just like carpal tunnel release surgery it doesn't always give complete relief. Since a surgical outcome can never be guaranteed, many experts consider surgery to be the last resort.

I underwent the surgery, but the pain in my feet never resolved. I may never have had tarsal tunnel syndrome in the first place. Such a pattern is typical of many people with FM who undergo unnecessary surgeries out of desperation, chasing the pain. After taking one month off I went back to work, where I was on my feet for eight hours a day. I was in constant pain, and I returned again and again to my podiatrist/surgeon. By now I wondered if the pain would ever stop.

Within a year additional symptoms manifested themselves. I was overcome with profound fatigue and pain in my upper and lower back, hips, and knees. I was frantic to find out what was happening to me. I had headaches every day. I wanted to sleep all the time, but I didn't feel refreshed when I got up in the morning. I stayed in the "keep it together; I will get better" mode as long as I could. My partner and I had just bought a house, so it was an awful time to quit working, especially since I couldn't predict when I might be able to work again. But finally I left my thirteen-year career as a florist.

About four months after leaving my job, I consulted another podiatrist. I was fed up with anti-inflammatories, icing my feet in five-gallon buckets of ice and water, and elevating them every moment they were not on the ground. Luckily, the new podiatrist was a colleague of a rheumatologist who specialized in fibromyalgia. I hardly remember the day when I met the rheumatologist and was diagnosed with FM. I am told that I cried all day when it began to sink in that this whole ordeal wasn't just the inability to heal after surgery, or a result of my being out of shape. I called my original podiatrist to let her know I had FM. She replied, "I always wondered if you did."

The fatigue brought on by my FM was so severe in those days it was all I could do to get to the store when I needed something. Then I'd be so exhausted from my outing that I couldn't even use the item I'd purchased till the next day. I remember lying on the sofa watching the first day of the O. J. Simpson trial. I thought, "Man, I really *am* sick if I am lying here watching this." Depression also hit me hard in those first few months. It lasted longer than a year while I came to terms with having a chronic illness. Then I began to take charge of my new life.

As the stories in this chapter indicate, other women have had experiences similar to mine—that of facing skeptical doctors, consulting with several specialists, or undergoing a battery of tests and treatments before finally getting diagnosed.

Gerry L. Once I was finally diagnosed, I was relieved that I was not crazy or dying. Still, the doctor called it "a wastepaper-basket diagnosis." He actually yelled at me because I couldn't tell him where my pain was. I yelled back, "It's all over!" He was finished doing tests to rule out other diseases, and I think he must have read something on fibromyalgia, so he said, "You have fibromyalgia." He didn't do a tender-point exam; he just said, "Take this medication and come back to see me in three or six months." I was frightened about what was happening to my body, yet he didn't explain anything to me about the condition. I saw him a few more times and then decided that I would no longer deal with him. I refuse to go to doctors who are unwilling to partner with me. The pain is in my body, not my head.

I later found out when I was gathering all my medical records that he'd never even documented that he'd said I had fibromyalgia. His nurse told me that since my ANA (antinuclear antibody) test was negative, I did not have fibromyalgia. I informed her that an ANA test was not the criterion for diagnosing fibromyalgia. I did go back later and give this nurse information about FM, which she welcomed, as her mother had just been diagnosed with it. I told her she had a wonderful opportunity to help other patients and to educate herself as well.

I am an R.N., and I have so often wondered how many nurses have FM. As women, we were raised to live up to the expectations of everyone else. We were the fixers, the ones trained to make everyone happy, the caregivers and nurturers. I know now that I emptied myself out. I had nothing left to give, especially for myself. I know people thought of me as the person who had it all together. Capable. With the perfect life.

Val T. I became ill with severe pain. My fingers were extremely painful, with burning and lack of coordination; it was very difficult to write. I also suffered from fever, body aches, fatigue, back pain, and irritable bowel syndrome. I think my being a nurse worked to my benefit, because the doctors I consulted took me seriously. My heart goes out to all those less fortunate. I was diagnosed with FM within three months by a rheumatologist who specialized in FM— but not until, of course, I underwent many blood tests and other tests to rule out everything else.

Along with probably every other FM patient, I've wondered why it is so difficult to get a diagnosis when statistics show that millions of people around the world have FM. The number of people diagnosed with the disorder continues to grow as people recognize themselves in media stories about FM. The good news is that doctors are becoming more aware of the syndrome and more willing to make the diagnosis. In 1999, the Social Security Administration officially recognized FM as a medically determined impairment, allowing people greater access to disability benefits. In addition, the American Medical Association, the American College of Rheumatology, the World Health Organization, and the National Institutes of Health all finally agree that FM is a legitimate illness.

The word *fibromyalgia* simply means "pain in the muscles, ligaments, and tendons." Fibromyalgia is referred to as a "syndrome" because it is characterized by a set of signs and symptoms that occur together. It is not a new syndrome. It has been around for over 150 years under different names such as *rheumatism* and *fibrositis*. Some of the women interviewed for this book received the diagnosis of fibrositis. According to the Fibromyalgia Network, "FM used to be called *fibrositis*, implying that there was inflammation in the muscles, but research later proved that inflammation did not exist." The Arthritis Foundation website, while clarifying that FM "is not a form of arthritis, nor is it associated with inflammation," classifies the condition as "a form of *soft-tissue rheumatism*, a broad term including a group of disorders that cause pain and stiffness around the joints and in the muscles and bones." *Rheumatologists* are specialists in musculoskeletal illnesses and immune disorders. Many FM patients rely on a rheumatologist as their primary health-care provider, and, as is the case with many FM'ers, it was a rheumatologist who finally made my diagnosis.

There are many illnesses of which pain and fatigue are the hallmark. In *Alternative Treatments for Fibromyalgia and Chronic Fatigue Syndrome* (ATF), Dr. Devin Starlanyl tells us that chronic myofascial pain syndrome is often confused with fibromyalgia and that people may have both conditions at once. (To add to the confusion, one medical encyclopedia written for home use identifies myofascial pain syndrome as a subcategory of fibromyalgia syndrome!) In this excerpt from her contribution to ATF, Dr. Starlanyl describes the physiological origins of myofascial pain syndrome and distinguishes it from fibromyalgia:

> Chronic myofascial pain syndrome is a condition of bodywide trigger points that are maintained by perpetuating factors, such as lack of sleep or poor sleep position.
>
> Most of us have seen the white, translucent covering on the muscles of chicken we buy at the grocery store. That is myofascia. The sticky covering wraps around bundles of muscle cells and around the muscles themselves. It interconnects throughout the whole body. Myofascia is very sticky stuff; it sticks together to form tendons and ligaments at the ends of muscles. When the

body experiences pain, the myofascia responds: the body reacts to pain immediately (because pain signifies damage), and the body goes into a self-protective stress mode. When this happens, the myofascia forms a sort of "splint," trying to minimize the pain by restricting movement. This "guarding" is part of the body's survival mechanism and is helpful on a short-term basis.

But when the pain becomes chronic and the guarding lasts, the muscle tightness inhibits the delivery of fuel and oxygen, as well as the removal of waste. An area of extreme sensitivity can develop. This is called a myofascial trigger point, and it is an area that is very painful when pressed and can refer pain and other symptoms in specific patterns throughout the body. When a muscle has trigger points it becomes weakened and shorter, and cannot stretch or do its normal job. It loses range of motion. Myofascial trigger points are not the same as the "tender points" found in FM patients, but they are neuromuscular in nature.

In myofascial pain syndrome, the muscle becomes hard as a rock. Often the trigger points can't be felt because of fluid in the muscles. Everything is very, very tight, and people may feel like they are wearing a wetsuit that is several sizes too small. Even the tightness itself can be painful.

Anyone can develop a myofascial trigger point, but if there are no perpetuating factors, it will become latent and won't cause symptoms unless it's activated (and if properly treated, it will go away). Perpetuating factors can include lack of sleep, pain, or certain body movements or positions. Even a poor sleeping position can be a perpetuating condition. Because these problems often accompany FM, people with FM are at special risk of developing myofascial pain syndrome. Although myofascial pain syndrome is not a progressive disorder, if you have a perpetuating factor such as FM and the trigger points are untreated or improperly treated, your body will soon develop a network of nodules and ropy bands....

People who have both FM and myofascial pain syndrome experience different problems from tender points and trigger points. FM's tender points can cause allover achiness. You can't have FM "in your back" or in your neck or hands. It's like saying you're "a little bit pregnant." You either have it all over or you don't. Myofascial trigger points, however, usually cause localized pain. FM also gives you the flulike feeling that never seems to let up. This fatigue is generally caused by lack of sleep.

⎽⎽⎽

In *Fibromyalgia and Chronic Myofascial Pain: A Survival Manual* (second edition), Dr. Starlanyl and Mary Ellen Copeland go into greater detail about the signs and symptoms of myofascial pain syndrome and trigger points. It is excellent material, with diagrams to help both you and your doctor or body worker understand where your pain is coming from and how best to treat it.

As stated in Chapter 1, the American College of Rheumatology has established that the following symptoms must coexist in order for an official diagnosis of FM to be made: widespread pain lasting three or more months and existing in all four quadrants of the body, plus pain in eleven out of eighteen tender-point sites. But not all medical practitioners agree with these criteria. Some believe that a person can have FM even if she or he doesn't meet the required number of tender points. Others question the reliability of tender points as a diagnostic tool. Even the experts are still learning about fibromyalgia! Therefore, it is important to tell your doctor about other, seemingly unrelated symptoms.

Nancy D. It took about three months for all the symptoms to show up and worsen. The first person to ever say the word fibromyalgia to me was my physical therapist, who has suffered from it for many years. I asked her a lot of questions because I could identify with what she said on every topic. Then my doctor directed me to the health and healing library, a local resource created specifically for patients. I couldn't get past the word fibromyalgia. I had to look it up many times. My education started through these healers, who pointed the way.

Ginger C. I was beginning to think I was losing it. It seemed like I was always finding some new ache or pain, and no apparent reason for them. Looking back now, I can see signs that I had FM probably as early as ten years ago, at least. I have always had frequent headaches, joint pain, and clumsiness.

⎽⎽⎽

Women have told me that prior to their diagnosis they failed to link the symptoms together. Their unrefreshing sleep, morning stiffness, and allover body pain seemed unrelated. My situation was the same; I had reasoned that my symptoms couldn't *all* be one illness. Additionally, so many strange things were happening in my body. Besides the inexplicable pain and fatigue, bright lights and loud sounds seemed like a physical assault on my body and brain. To someone with FM, such everyday phenomena can be perceived as pain. On one occasion before my diagnosis, my partner banged on the hood of a car I was sitting in. Even though she did it simply to announce her presence, it startled me so that I was flooded with a wave of anxiety and emotion. I cried all the way home. When you have FM, it is hard to make your loved ones understand the ways in which your body has become foreign to you.

At the same time, it is essential to accurately and thoroughly describe your pain, fatigue, and other symptoms to your doctor—only then can he or she ultimately determine whether you have FM. First, however, find a doctor who knows how to treat FM and who believes that he or she can help you. Adopt the attitude that you're looking for a partner in healing. (Read Chapter 9 for more about dealing with doctors and other medical professionals.) A good source for finding doctors and other practitioners is through a local FM support group. There, you can meet women who might be able to suggest a doctor who is well educated in FM and has an open attitude. The Arthritis Foundation hotline can lead you to a support group in your area (see Resources).

Jean T.   When I finally got a doctor to confirm that I did have fibromyalgia, I was beginning to think I must be losing my mind. I think I had FM for at least five years before anyone finally said it was a legitimate illness and that I wasn't malingering. One of my sons actually said I was only doing this for sympathy because I had to take care of his father. The terrible thing is that now he also has a chronic condition and is unable to work. He doesn't talk to me, so I can't find out for sure what his status is.

I have been diagnosed for about seven years. I know it all started when I had the flu. My doctor has agreed he thinks it started with a virus. My doctor is wonderful—he looks like George Clooney. (I told you I am not old! Anyway, my sister says that after a certain number of years, you can say outrageous things to good-looking men, as long as you remain a lady.) Aside from being good-looking, he is a great doctor. He always says he wishes he could do more for me and that he is in it with me.

After being diagnosed with FM, I began to have other bizarre symptoms. Lack of balance was the worst one, until a tremor started in my left hand. That sent me running to the doctor. After a whole battery of tests, including two MRIs, I was told that in addition to the fibromyalgia, I also have a rare Parkinsonian-like condition known as multiple systems atrophy (MSA). I was also told that before it is over I will be in a wheelchair.

I have done a lot of research on the Internet, and I feel I have a pretty good understanding of both illnesses. I am more or less holding my own with both of them.

Sisu G.   In my case the process of arriving at a diagnosis was a gradual one. I was very fortunate in that I was dealing with open, earnest doctors. (I did have one doctor who was filling in for my primary-care physician and who wouldn't listen, so I switched to another doctor within the same system.) My initial problems were not with pain but rather with my breathing, a complication caused by my celiac disease (a genetic intolerance to gluten), which was also undiagnosed at the time. Eventually, besides my breathing problems, I couldn't fight off colds, I was tired all the time, my hands hurt, and I felt very weak. After being treated with asthma medication for the breathing issues, I switched hospitals and was put in the care of a physician who didn't know what to make of me. I lacked health insurance at the time, so I had to keep working. I switched to office work from retail because I was no longer able to stand for extended periods. I was finally tested for celiac disease when my sister was diagnosed with it. Soon afterwards, we found that eliminating wheat and a lot of other gluten-containing foods from my diet eased some of my symptoms.

I was sent to a neurologist. At no time did he treat me as if this were an imaginary illness. I received prompt and thorough medical care, including an awful lot of examinations, MRIs, and EMGs (electromyograms). I was being tested for MS, for lupus—for a number of awful diseases. The neurologist was very careful to examine every aspect of what could be causing my pain and numbness; he even examined me for tender points. I kept getting worse all the time. When no ready cause for my symptoms appeared on the neurological front, he said he wanted me to visit the rheumatology department. I was more than happy to cooperate. The rheumatologist told me I most likely had fibromyalgia, and after examining me and checking my blood tests once again to rule out lupus, he gave me a firm diagnosis. He has been very solid in his assurances that this is a real, albeit mysterious, ailment, and he's urged me to find out all I can about it.

I had experienced some symptoms, such as morning pain and sleep twitches, for more than five years before my diagnosis. No one is quite sure at what point the symptoms became severe and numerous enough to cross the line into FM, so I would have to say that I had full-blown FM for only about a year and a half before my diagnosis. As soon as the symptoms became intense enough to point out to a doctor, it took about three months to come to a diagnosis.

Because all my doctors had been so open, I was not shocked or surprised by the diagnosis. They told me it was easier to be open with a patient who was taking initiative, i.e., asking questions, bringing in notes, paying attention. I didn't know much about the illness, so it did feel unreal, but for the most part I experienced a wave of sincere relief to know that I wasn't going to end up in a wheelchair at twenty-five. Earlier, I remember sitting at home and saying that celiac disease was the best diagnosis I could have received, because it wasn't fatal and could be treated. And I remember thinking the same about FM. If I get to choose, I want FM rather than MS or lupus, because at least this one gives me a chance; it is a condition to manage, not merely to try to avoid dying from. I wouldn't trade it for some of the other illnesses I could have. I keep this firmly in mind on my bad days.

Getting a firm diagnosis has done me a great deal of good. Now I know I'm not going to die. I know if I choose carefully, I can do a few of the activities I need and want to do—and that gives me some sense of control. My lifestyle is profoundly limited, and there is nothing that prepares one for the grief that settles in when the reality of not being able to participate in normal life becomes clear. That's a real issue for me, and one I deal with every day. But if I am careful, I can skip doing laundry and go to a movie. I have to measure very carefully how I feel.

Cydney B. I had no idea what FM was. Eight years ago, when I had been treated for rheumatoid arthritis for two years, the rheumatologist sort of offhandedly mentioned fibromyalgia when I asked why my muscles, as well as my joints, felt sore. I went home and looked up the word. It sounded a lot less threatening to me at that point than the RA. The rheumatologist seemed to treat it as a side issue and did not offer any treatment at that point. I thought it was a nuisance, but not much more than that. The RA is now mostly in remission.

No one has really concluded whether FM has a prodrome (a symptom that offers a premonition of a disease) or a genetic defect, or if it lies smoldering for years until it finally becomes a big enough issue that the sufferer seeks medical care. I had the usual growing pains as a child, mostly in my legs. When I was a single mother in my thirties, I experienced what I would call "lost weekends." About four times a year I would come home on Friday from a week of work, go to bed so exhausted that I could barely move, and sleep almost nonstop until Sunday at about six P.M. I'd get up to feed the kids and check on them periodically, but I was pretty well out cold all weekend. Then I'd sleep a normal night's sleep and go back to work. In my mid-thirties I went to a few doctors complaining of terrible pain in my upper back between my shoulder blades. The pain would be present for weeks, then go away for maybe a year or more, and then come back. I was told—and actually believed—that women my age often complained of similar back pain and that it was just part of being an "overachiever." I had a very good job, was a single mother of two accomplished young children, and thus evidently an overachiever, a label I heard repeatedly thereafter and very specifically at the time of my diagnosis with rheumatoid arthritis. In 1991, at age forty-three, I had a car accident. Within months I started having hip pain, for which I sought treatment. I had not injured my hip in the accident. My condition sort of rolled downhill from there.

So I fit the usual medical history of someone with FM. The Mayo Clinic pronounced me a "classic case" of fibromyalgia, with the classic history.

▲▲▲

Don't let any challenges and resistance you may have encountered in dealing with health-care professionals—and possibly even from your loved ones—deter you from getting to the bottom of what is wrong with you. Accurate diagnosis of FM (or any other chronic condition) is the first step in learning to live well with it. Put your fears aside and get on with finding the origin of your pain and fatigue.

THE RELIEF OF A DIAGNOSIS

Charlene M. I was grateful that now I could put a name to what was wrong with me and that I wasn't out of my mind.

Kay B. I was greatly relieved when I was told exactly what was wrong with me. My eclectic group of symptoms did not fit any other condition, and I was beginning to think they were all in my head!

Diane H. I felt relieved. I finally had something with a name and a description. I had been going to my doctor for five to ten years with various aches, pains, and other symptoms, and he could never find anything "wrong." I would greet him with, "Here I am, your favorite middle-aged hypochondriac." He would assure me that I wasn't a hypochondriac. One time I responded, "But you're one of the finest diagnosticians in Phoenix, so either I'm a hypochondriac or you're a shitty doctor!"

There is great relief for patients in learning that FM is a real illness, a medical syndrome. Millions live with it all over the world. FM is not "in your head." Within the last ten years FM has been the subject of many books and media reports, and it seems as though everyone knows someone who has it. Many women have told me of their relief at finally finding out what was causing them years of pain, fatigue, headache, and stiffness. In response to my survey question about how they felt upon being diagnosed with FM, women overwhelmingly reported feeling relief.

But the sense of relief typically isn't untainted, for equally as often the respondents to my survey reported feeling shock and fear. As Sisu points out above, there's no escaping the grief that accompanies the realization that your life might be severely limited for who knows how long by this chronic, debilitating illness. As bewildered and frustrated as you feel before being diagnosed— when you're grappling with a bunch of mysterious, incapacitating symptoms-without-a-name, until a definite label is pinned on your condition—you might nurture a small hope that one morning you'll wake up and the symptoms will have disappeared, as inexplicably as they arrived. Receiving the news that you have a chronic disorder with no known cure, while reassuring, is at the same time devastating.

Right after my own diagnosis, because I knew the basics about FM, I was afraid! My emotions came out as anxiety, anger, and depression, but really I was just scared. I didn't understand FM's cycle, what medications to try, or what to do about the unrelenting pain. I started searching for answers. Joining a support group helped me to understand that now, as soon as possible after diagnosis, was the time to find out as much as I could about FM. (For an in-depth discussion of the depression, anger, and other strong emotions that can accompany fibromyalgia, see Chapter 6.)

Gina H. When I was first told I had FM, I had never heard of it. When the doctor explained the condition to my husband and me, I felt afraid, because the doctor didn't seem to have any kind of expression on his face that I could identify with. I stopped hearing and started reading his face, and what I read was that there was no cure for the illness nor any clue as to how I got it. Once I started listening again, I heard these words: "The only thing I can do is make you comfortable." I just knew then that I was getting ready to die, and I was angry with the doctor, with my husband, and with my heavenly father.

Val T. I felt relieved when I finally received my diagnosis! I was so afraid it was rheumatoid arthritis; I believed that would have been devastating. Little did I know how bad FM really was. I knew very little about it, so I started doing tons of research. I tried very hard to exercise because I knew it would help. I concentrated on sleep.

Then my emotions went on a roller-coaster ride. I was afraid my husband would not want me anymore. I was very mad that I'd become ill, and also uncertain about the future and about my employment and continuing my career. I blamed my illness on my work at the clinic. It seemed every nurse who has worked there has grown ill with some condition like FM, rheumatoid arthritis, chronic fatigue syndrome, Crohn's disease, autoimmune disorders, hypothyroidism, Hashimoto's thyroiditis, irritable bowel syndrome, or multiple sclerosis. After my diagnosis I started researching how many health-care professionals get FM or CFS, and I have found that a very high number do—with the highest numbers among nurses! Is this because our immune systems are continually bombarded with infectious illnesses? Would I be well if I'd never worked as a nurse? I have no concrete answers, but I do know there are many of us afflicted. A young nurse at my clinic just came down with chronic fatigue syndrome recently, after working there for less than a year!

Thinking back, I guess I never wanted to accept my diagnosis. I was in denial, and to this day I still am when I have my pain under control. I hate the word fibromyalgia! Lately, when I'm pain-free, I try to convince everyone that I no longer have anything wrong with me. However, the pain in my back when the caudal (an epidural injection to treat back pain) wears off is a rude awakening that I was only fooling myself. Before FM, I was always extremely healthy. I wouldn't even admit to having a cold.

Donna F. I felt rather hopeless when I was diagnosed with fibromyalgia. I was told there was no cure—that you just have to find a way to manage the pain through diet, exercise, medications, massage therapy, acupuncture, hot packs, cold packs, hot tubs, and/or any other means available. These forms of management for the most part are expensive and time-consuming. The news was especially discouraging because of the demands on me as a mother of four, one of whom has significant special needs.

Rachel B. At first I was relieved, but shortly afterward I was angry. No treatment protocol was in place, and only the symptoms could be treated. I was unsure about the extent of impact it would have upon my own and my partner's life. Going from doing triathlons, mountaineering, mountain biking, sea lifeguarding, and waterskiing to a much different type of physical exertion such as yoga or archery is hard to accept, especially when you are used to pushing your body to the limit. Now, just getting through a day of work can be a challenge at times.

Donnie M. I was actually relieved to finally receive a correct diagnosis and happy to know I did not have polymyalgia rheumatica, as originally diagnosed by my primary-care physician a year earlier. By now I'd found a rheumatologist at UCLA in Los Angeles. It was good to be seeing a specialist who was kind, compassionate, and knowledgeable about my condition. It was good to hear him say he would work with me to get me off the prednisone I had been taking since being misdiagnosed with polymyalgia rheumatica; I'd felt it was going to kill me with all its side effects. After he had evaluated and examined me, his words to me were, "You do not have polymyalgia, and you never should have been put on prednisone. You have fibromyalgia. The good news is it will not kill you, but the bad news is there will be times when you wish it would." My reply was, "I already know about those times."

Everything in my life has changed, even the clothes I am able to wear. My feeling is that the FM is now in charge, not me, and that I can only do what the FM will allow me to do. If I ever dare to try and take control from this ugly beast, I get knocked down and end up in bed with a major flare-up. I no longer have much of a life; I just exist. This monster that no one understands is something I lack the ability to fight.

WHAT TO DO AFTER YOUR DIAGNOSIS

Your next step is to find others who live with FM. They can hold you up during the early days after diagnosis, when just talking about FM—that is, connecting with people who share the same day-to-day pain and fatigue—helps so much. Through my doctor, I found a support group right after I was diagnosed. I called it the FM Mutiny Group, because after a while the core six of us drifted away from the larger group and began to meet in our homes.

If you live in a small town where no groups are already formed, consider trying to start one yourself, or at least a phone tree. Do this by hanging a sign at the grocery store or any other place that hosts a community bulletin board.

Most groups in my area are large enough to attract good speakers and to have moderators who organize the subjects put up for the night's discussion. Sometimes it's an open meeting, when members can share. Those occasions are valuable. You will hear about people's experiences with new medications and treatments, new doctors in the area, and ways for coping with FM.

Sometimes I think support groups have a reputation of people sitting around complaining about their lives. In fact, support groups usually encourage attendees to focus on the solution rather than the problem. Our group meetings have been the source of interesting, educational, and useful information. I have never left a meeting feeling less than optimistic about something new. And I have made some good friends in support groups.

Gerry L. Only in a support group can you feel what others are going through. As we discuss and share, we comfort each other. We know because we've been there.

Nancy D. My doctor referred me to the Arthritis Foundation to find a support group. Since there were no support groups for the weird diseases my doctor mentioned and since I had all the symptoms of FM/CFS, I went to that support group. Every meeting I attended resulted in knowledge or the ability to obtain knowledge that supports my health every day. When I moved back to Washington state, I attended a similar group one time. There were only three other attendees, and one guy who couldn't find the Depressed Anonymous meeting, so he joined in on ours. It was at that meeting that the group leader showed us your first book *(Alternative Treatments for Fibromyalgia and Chronic Fatigue Syndrome)*. I bought it and took it everywhere and even discussed it with my doctors.

▲▲▲

For Renee Wilkins, being a support-group member evolved into being a support-group leader. This role has brought unexpected rewards to her life with FM. Here are her comments:

1984: New job as a national sales trainer. New mentor: Ira. New quest: self-awareness. Biggest lesson I have to learn: "Unconditional love for self and others." What does he mean by that?

1987: The happiest and saddest year of my life. I was a new bride of three months. I was exposed to industrial chemicals, and then came the diagnosis of FM/CFS. What is that? My personality began to change. What is happening to me?

1988: Terminated from my job. Had to rely on long-term disability and Social Security disability.

1989: My doctor suggested a support group. Oh well, what could it hurt? I found help and a place to be me as I was—sick, tired, and out of hope. But I also found more. I found people who listened, understood, and became friends and confidants. I could see them once a month and feel hope and learn to cope with this disease, whatever it was.

I learned about the grieving process, about denial and acceptance, pacing, and other life skills for survival. I found several mentors who'd had this illness for ten years or longer. I listened, learned, and bargained with God for a cure or at least a higher state of well-being. I learned that it was my choice to be or not be ill. The choice I had to make was this: What am I willing to do to get to a higher state of well-being?

My support-group leader, friend, and mentor asked me for help in running the group. Most of the members had already taken a turn at running the group. Was it my turn? I had made progress; could I make more by helping others? The experienced members said being involved makes you focus on the things you most need to do to get to that higher state of well-being. I helped a little. Would no one else step forward to become the new group leader? There were others healthier than I, but their decisions were to get back to life as much as possible. They wanted to relate to the healthy world. I bargained with God—if I do this, will you heal me? I took the leap of faith. I needed to restore my self-esteem, my sense of self, a way to find out about the newest treatments and to be connected to something bigger than myself.

I have been a support-group leader for ten years now. I know God doesn't bargain for good health if we promise to do good works. I know he answers prayers, but in his time, not ours. Being a support-group leader has taught me the most important lesson of my life: unconditional love for myself and others.

I'm a support-group leader because it makes me feel needed and because it is a scale upon which I can judge my improvement. I enjoy all the warm, fuzzy feelings the groups give me. The hugs, the calls, the thank-you cards. A stroke for my ego? You bet. Why not?

Some FM'ers have found support online:

Val T. There are no support groups for FM in the area where I live, but last spring I joined an online FM/CFS support group (at www.ImmuneSupport.com). As a nurse, I try to help many of the group members, as well as describing which of the therapies I've tried work and which don't. Everyone is very supportive. They have been there with kind words many times when I have been down. They have taught me a lot as well. It is a very large group, and new members join on a daily basis. A couple of the forum moderators are key to the group's success. They keep it safe from salesmen, and they also direct postings to different message boards that are more appropriate.

Sisu G. I have a group of friends who all belong to an online community that I put together for posting to them about my condition and group events and so on. There is a bulletin board that I visit when I really need to ask other people about how they cope. My rheumatologist is definitely part of my support network, because he's a big help.

Penny G. I am a member of two Yahoo groups concerning FM. I have occasionally attended local support groups. There is an excellent one that meets about twenty-five miles from my location, but it conflicts with my work schedule. I also know two women locally with FM whom I can talk to. I have a few girlfriends with their own health issues who are pretty understanding.

I don't feel accepted by most FM groups because I am still able to do quite a bit. I think some people with FM resent the fact that my illness has not progressed as far as theirs has. I get better support when I am going through a flare, because then they can relate to me. Healthy people do not understand my struggles at all.

Donnie M. My one and only support comes from the WebMD computer site. I chat sometimes and always keep up with the message board. These fellow FM friends are my lifeline. I learn from them, feel I can be myself, and certainly know they are the only ones who truly understand the hell I live in. I cried the first time I found this site. I said to my husband, "They are there and they understand." It was absolutely wonderful to know someone else had this illness and actually understood!

▲▲▲

Consider also seeking guidance from a trained mental-health professional familiar with FM. A person wouldn't think twice about seeking a therapist if she had just been diagnosed with lupus or MS. FM should be no different. The diagnosis of any chronic illness can bring on feelings of loss, depression, anxiety, and despair.

If you haven't done so already, find a doctor who will be your partner in learning to live with FM. Make sure this provider understands and believes that FM is a real illness, worthy of his or her time. It might take a few visits and doctor changes to find the person best suited to manage your illness, but the time is well spent. You may end up with a rheumatologist, a general practitioner, a naturopathic physician, or a chiropractor. It is up to you to find the best fit.

After talking to many women living with fibromyalgia, I've concluded that those who manage their illness holistically seem to have the best results. There is no cure for FM—yet. Diet, exercise, lifestyle changes, medications, supplements, and support are the mainstay of a sound program to live a better life with FM.

Nancy D. It has been a constant challenge to find ways to comfort myself. One way I have discovered is to take a role in my own health. My idea of an illness prior to this whole ordeal was to go to the doctor, have him make a diagnosis and prescribe a pill, and hope that in a few days I would feel better.

△△△

A few of my FM friends have recovered enough to go to school and/or get a job. In my support group, my dear friend Ellen J. seemed to be the most ill of all of us. She has FM, chronic multiple chemical sensitivity (MCS), arthritis, chronic fatigue syndrome (CFS), and sleep apnea. It took at least eight years of changing her lifestyle and her living space and really working hard on getting better, but Ellen recovered enough to return to college and finish her degree. She did it by going about her recovery very methodically. She read everything she could find on FM, CFS, and MCS. She educated herself and her doctors. She created a "safe" home without toxic cleaners and cosmetics, and she was strict with the people around her. She adjusted her diet and adhered to a daily exercise program. She found the right combination of medications that worked for her. Bit by bit, over time, her symptoms lessened enough for her to continue her education. But to me, the greatest part of Ellen's healing came the day she decided that FM wouldn't be number one in her life. She decided not to respond to her symptoms in an emotionally negative way. At that point, a shift took place. FM may or may not be a lifelong condition, but once Ellen's symptoms were addressed, she was able to focus on the rest of her life.

The lesson we can take from Ellen's story is this: Your diagnosis is just the beginning. Now it's time to find out all you can about how best to live with this illness. Make doing so your number-one priority. There is no magic pill and no doctor who can "fix" it. Doctors can point the way, but ultimately it is you who must discover how to live well with FM. It is your body, after all. No one knows FM better than you do. To help you in your journey, later chapters in this book offer stories of how women deal with the chronic pain, fatigue, and other symptoms of FM.

Also remember another important lesson Ellen learned: FM is part of you, but it is not you.

The Unique Concerns of Women with FM

All the statistics agree that women are diagnosed with fibromyalgia much more often than men. But the question remains why that's so. No definitive answer exists to this mystery, but some people believe it may have as much to do with societal conditioning—that is, with differences in how the sexes perceive and report pain and illness—as it does with physiology. This issue is explored in the first part of this chapter.

You'll also hear from our community of correspondents regarding other matters of special interest to women living with FM: how the illness can affect menstruation and menopause (and vice versa), its impact on sexual intimacy, dealing with FM and thyroid problems (another condition for which women are at greater risk than men), and the possible benefits and risks of hormone replacement therapy. The chapter closes with reflections from a few women on what they've learned about themselves *as women* from this illness.

WHY MORE WOMEN?

Statistics vary as to the ratio of women versus men who are diagnosed with FM. *The New Sjögren's Syndrome Handbook* reports that the overall prevalence of FM in the U.S. population is 2 percent, with 3.4 percent of these cases occurring in women and 0.5 percent of these cases occurring in men. The American College of Rheumatology website states that FM occurs seven times more frequently in women than in men.

Although experts have not yet established any conclusive answer about why so many more women than men contract this illness, some have linked the issue to hormonal imbalances. In my earlier book, *Alternative Treatments for Fibromyalgia and Chronic Fatigue Syndrome* (ATF), Carol Landis, D.N.Sc., of the University of Washington, reports that women FM patients whom she has studied "have considerably reduced amounts of growth hormone compared to our age-matched controls." Other researchers have also made the connection between FM and inadequate levels of growth hormone (which is necessary in adults for tissue repair and regulation of metabolism). The Fibromyalgia Network states, "At least one-third of FM patients meet the criteria for adult growth hormone deficiency." (For more about growth hormone and FM, see Kim Dupree-Jones's comments in Chapter 12.) Interestingly, Landis and her colleagues also found, "quite unexpectedly," that women with FM have reduced levels of prolactin, a pituitary hormone important in lactation.

And then there's a theory regarding serotonin levels and another theory centered around a possible autoimmune component of FM. Patricia S., an M.D. and one of our community of FM'ers, offers her ideas along these lines:

Patricia S. Serotonin is one of the many, many regulators of pain in the body. Women have a very different serotonin profile from men. We have less serotonin in our bodies, which is the same reason why women are more often depressed. Maybe, too, fibromyalgia has an autoimmune component to it, because a lot of women with autoimmune problems also have fibromyalgia. Why do women get more autoimmune diseases than men? It has something to do with how the immune system of women differs from that of men. Why is our immune system different? We don't know, but we think it might have something to do with the design of the female body for childbirth, how the body regulates the whole reproductive system and has to deal with this foreign object in it called a baby. We are not just men with vaginas. Ours is a whole different framework, like the desert is different from the Olympia National Park rainforest. They're both on the earth and they both have trees and land, but their terrain is very different.

Other members of our FM community speculate as follows on the question of a physiological basis for the difference between the incidence of FM in women and men (be aware that these individuals are not medical professionals, but rather laypeople. Their opinions must be regarded with that fact in mind):

Victoria M. I think hormones are the basis for FM being largely a female illness. The metabolic characteristics of women are very different from those of men. I believe the biochemistry that supports hormonal metabolism is similarly deficient in men; however, the greater needs of women due to the menstrual cycle, the childbearing years, and even the menopausal years exacerbates the condition in women.

Sisu G. There may be biological differences—especially in the HPA (hypothalamus, pituitary, and adrenal glands) axis and in the way the hormones are balanced—that contribute to this illness being more of a female issue.

Diane H. I think there may be a hormonal factor involved, because when I finally started using progesterone cream instead of antidepressants, my depression resolved.

To find out how women perceive themselves in this so-called women's illness, I asked them to tell me why they think seven out of ten FM patients are female. Many of the respondents tended to fall into two general camps: women who believe they cope differently from men with regard to illness and pain and those who don't see any clear gender-based differences. Below are some women's answers to this question:

Charlene M. I think a man would have a harder time and take longer to seek help and then take even longer to make himself rest when he needs to in order to ease into a flare.

Sonia H. I saw a television interview with a man and a woman who had recently been diagnosed with chronic fatigue syndrome, and he was not accepting of it. He was railing against it, he was angry, he was irritated and impatient, he was trying to figure out how to live with it or how to solve some of the problems, and he was just mad. I don't know if that is typical of other men who have chronic illnesses, but I think in general they don't have as much patience with being ill as women do.

Cybill C. I think I definitely cope differently as a woman. Men tend to internalize their feelings and to be more hesitant to seek medical care.

Victoria M. I think men tend to tough things out. They are less likely to seek treatment, less likely to take vitamins, less likely to change their lifestyle and habits willingly, less likely to accept the condition, and less likely to get the help they need. I think the role of financial provider would make it very stressful to change circumstances, because of all the conditioning and perceptions about being male. And in this illness, one has to change.

I know through my own dealings with men that they suffer and take a long time to build a rapport that allows them to trust and be willing to listen and make changes that may benefit them. They are not used to being helpless and unable to control life's outcomes.

Whereas I will seek answers through intuition and faith, I have found that men need to have evidence and reasoning to make changes. I think we all cope differently, and I think it is very hard for men. We women know the pain of childbirth, etc., but fewer men have had to deal with intense pain.

Emma L. I have learned that I am very strong and have a basic "philosophy of life." I do not think it makes any difference that I am a woman, but this is cultural, as the split between men and women is not so pronounced in Italy as it is in the United States. I do not think that a man or a woman copes differently. A lot is based on societal expectations, and having changed countries freed me of most of those demands. I also personally do not believe that women and men are different. I have been lucky enough to have known a few men very, very well and to establish that they are no different from women.

Sondra H.   It's hard to say that I cope with FM differently than a man would. FM can be so different in people. Some suffer greatly, others mildly. People have varying levels of pain tolerance. Coping is something very personal, because of each person's individuality and mindset.

▲▲▲

In the last few years, I have met quite a few men who live with FM. I have met them online, at support groups, and through family. I interviewed several men for my first book, ATF, and found that men deal with FM just as we women do, one day at a time. They modify their lives so it is easier to complete tasks, make their working space or office as ergonomic as possible, and do everything they can for pain. Additionally, all of the men I have met use exercise as an important part of their pain-control regime. David A. wrote the following about coming to terms with FM:

> I did yoga daily in an effort to loosen up. I also had much less tolerance for sitting down for long periods. My attention span decreased, too. I left work in February 1995....
>
> My life has definitely changed a lot since I got sick. I used to go backpacking or cross country skiing every weekend or every other weekend...but we don't do that much now. I worked for Microsoft as a programmer, but now I can't even type anymore. I was a musician, a drummer, and I can't do that anymore, either. Those are the main compromises I've made.
>
> I was very strongly linked to my physical activities, mentally and physically; they represented who I was as a person. I've had to totally redefine that and place less emphasis on my physical abilities.... One of the hardest lessons to learn is that I am not my body.

▲▲▲

Another important aspect of how women perceive the difference between women's and men's experiences of FM has to do with the sexes' respective relationships with the health-care establishment:

Victoria M. I think women are more likely to seek help, although I think men are more likely to get help when they seek it. I think men are more likely to have insurance policies that cover illness, and thus they are less likely to be financially dependent on others. I think doctors respect men more than women and would be more supportive and helpful if a man presented with these symptoms. Illness in men is more credible than illness in women. It is always our hormones!

Diane H. Most men don't report aches and pains or depression to their doctors as often as women do, if they even go to their doctors.

Sisu G. Women are encouraged in this culture to report pains to doctors, to examine pain, and to seek answers. Men are generally discouraged from seeking medical help for non-life-threatening ailments. Men are also less encouraged to compare experiences, which means that women may tend to have a better general view of how much pain is reasonable to tolerate and when to accept that it's a problem. So I would say that the answer to why so many more FM patients are women is partly medical and partly skewed by issues of patient–doctor communication, publicly held views of pain and illness, and publicly held views on gender-appropriate ailments and complaints.

Sisu's comments hit upon one more issue in the sexes' different experiences of FM: societal gender roles. Below are more observations on this topic:

Diane H. Women tend to be caregivers and overachievers with multiple roles that stress them into getting FM.

Victoria M. I think men get the chance to rest more readily than women do.

Norah T. As a woman, I learned to not identify my pain. I had work to do, I had kids to raise, and if I hurt, I hurt. On that level, I wasn't in denial. I knew it was there and I discussed it with the doctor whenever I went in, but the reality was, I was a single mom with four kids.

In *Alternative Treatments for Fibromyalgia and Chronic Fatigue Syndrome*, Tom O. reflects on societal expectations of men and how this affects coping with illness:

I really wonder, though, if they would understand. I think part of it is that macho-man thing. If I said, "Hey man, I've got FM and I'm feeling like hell today," maybe they would look at me like, Huh? Women can call up their friends, have a little get-together, and talk about this stuff: "What do you do and how do you get help and blah blah blah." I envy that about women. For a man, though, it's different. We all complain. But we don't really talk about it. We just go on.

Gina's story, which follows, emphasizes what so many of us know firsthand: As women we are expected—and we expect ourselves—to be available for everybody else, no matter what.

Gina H. I believe FM affects so many more women because we were Superwomen. We did it all. We worked, we took the kids to school, games, movies, over to friends' houses. My son has a friend who lived over a hundred miles away, and I would make the trip to their house and back. I bought the groceries, cooked, and then washed the dishes. I shopped for my family's clothes, including my husband's, washed them, put them away, and paid the bills, shuffling them to see who we were going to pay and who could wait until next week. I sat up with the kids when they were sick and took off work for doctor visits. This is where the stress came in. If any of the millions of ladies who have this disease thought they were Superwomen, they know what I am talking about. We just kept giving until we couldn't give any more.

▲▲▲

When we women make it a priority to put our health and well-being first, we open the door to the possibility of leading a more balanced and healthful life.

MENSTRUATION, MENOPAUSE, AND FM

One of the major ways that fibromyalgia impacts women is by affecting the very hormonal patterns that most define us as women: our menstrual cycles and our experience of peri-menopause and menopause. Many respondents to my survey reported that their periods became heavier and/or more painful after the onset of FM and that PMS symptoms became more pronounced. The inverse occurs, too: Menstruation can cause an increase in FM-related symptoms. Likewise, some women observed that the approach of menopause—and menopause itself—impacted their FM.

As for myself, my body has changed tremendously with the onset of FM. The flow of my periods is heavier, and the cycle lasts longer. Before FM, my period lasted for three days. Now I sometimes have it for five days or more, plus spotting for a few days, too.

PMS is a reality for many women, not a joke. When I have PMS, I mostly want to sleep and eat carbohydrates. In addition, anger—rage, really—builds up in me until my period begins, and then a physical and mental calming, a release, takes over. I blame the loss of five Fiestaware plates and several saucers on a recent menstrual cycle. While I'm menstruating, to help me view my period as something positive, I try to imagine all the toxins flowing out of me.

My FM pain increases dramatically during the week leading up to my period and during my period itself, and then I have two weeks of "normal" FM pain. I also seem to retain fluid, enough to cause five to eight pounds of weight gain just before my period.

My abdomen feels tight and uncomfortable, and my leg pain increases.

Lindamarie M. When my menstrual flow begins, it is painful, both vaginally and abdominally. My flow is heavier than ever since the onset of FM; I need two double-thick pads! My moods are beyond reason. I've tried numerous estrogen supplements and creams to help me find sanity, yet they just made me flow off the charts.

Norah T. I hit puberty at fourteen. The symptoms I now know as fibromyalgia started at age ten, and that actually could have been an onset due to prepubertal hormonal changes. But there was no way to identify that, because there was no before and after. There was nobody who knew what was going on.

My FM got worse by the time I reached menopause, which began early for me. Who knows if that had a relationship to the fibromyalgia? I reached menopause by forty-six, after which I had more pain across the board, unqualified. It was wicked. The increased level of pain still hasn't completely gone away, even now that I am sixty-one.

Katie G. FM does impact my menstrual cycle. Each month, a week or so prior to the onset of my cycle, my symptoms of profound fatigue, joint and muscle ache, headache, loss of balance, lack of concentration, cognitive difficulties, and flulike symptoms heighten. I often refer to them as being demonic. I need to nap more and longer. It is as if my body were operated via battery power, and I suddenly lost almost all power. I just stop and have to go to bed. I can't even talk or think. This has happened during all phases of my cycle, but especially a week before and during. I also find that I drop items or they fall out of my hand, as if the signal from my brain to my hand got cut or disconnected.

Cybill C. My menstrual flow has become much heavier since the onset of FM, and I tend to suffer PMS symptoms for two weeks instead of my usual one week.

SEXUAL RELATIONSHIPS

A serious illness such as FM can bring with it upsetting changes in one's sex life. Pain and the effects of prescription meds may put a damper on sexual desire. Self-esteem—and with it feelings of sexual attractiveness—can suffer when you're diagnosed with a debilitating illness. Working toward getting your health back may leave little energy left over for sex.

My partner and I try our best to enjoy a full sexual relationship, but often pain and fatigue get in the way of lovemaking. One way we work to enhance intimacy is to remember to communicate well; that way, when it's time to be close, our everyday problems don't go upstairs and into bed with us.

Other tips that work for us include keeping the lights low, having lots of pillows on hand for comfort, and beginning with massage and light touching. A soft massage seems to slow down the pain enough for my libido to kick in.

Orgasm isn't always the reason to make love. For people with chronic pain, sometimes having an orgasm isn't possible, due to side effects from medication or overwhelming pain or fatigue. Touching, talking together quietly, or being held might be all we can do on some days. Remind your partner that his or her happiness is important to you, but you may not always be able to include yourself in the end result. Remember, too, that in addition to the libido-diminishing effects of chronic pain, many drugs can cause a person to lose the desire for sex.

With all these factors potentially affecting the sexuality of someone with FM, it might be tempting to let the sexual part of your relationship "slide." But lovemaking can increase endorphins—raising our spirits and boosting our overall sense of well-being—and can help us feel closer to our partners, so it's worth doing all you can to avoid missing out on this very important part of a loving relationship. Honest, kind communication between partners can work as an effective aphrodisiac. Talk about sex together, try to come to an understanding of your partner's needs, and speak up about your own.

Cybill C. My relationship with my husband changed a lot. Our sex life became minimal, due to my fatigue and pain. Resentment built up because he didn't understand and didn't believe I was sick.

Penny G. There are some sexual issues, as I am in pain and rarely "in the mood." I try to be sexual when I can, so I feel bad when I am hardly ever sexual. My husband says he loves me and that he is not really concerned. I find it hard to believe him.

Lindamarie M. When making love, I try to go with the flow. If my legs are doing well, I usually get in the "on top" position; otherwise, being on the bottom helps me through any pain or swelling in my legs or ankles. Keeping my legs up helps with the painful stabbing I get in my legs and feet, and in turn the relief from pain helps me to enjoy sexual relations. Sometimes just saying the word sex exhausts me. Before FM, I shared a terrific sex life with my spouse.

As a woman, since my diagnosis I've learned how much I appreciate moments when I can shave, bathe, or even put on makeup. These simple daily tasks are such an effort to do today, and I did not appreciate them before my diagnosis. I took it all for granted. Even exercising to feel good and look good and dancing to allow the sexual being in me to come alive—I pray to have these simple things back in my womanly life!

SEXUAL INTIMACY AND PAIN

I experience pain with penetration, as well as exterior genital pain, called *vulvodynia*, and I've never known why. These symptoms have become worse with the onset of FM. Vulvodynia involves a burning, itching pain, similar to a severe abrasion on the skin. As you can imagine, my sexual life has been limited due to pain, both the vaginal pain and the muscular pain of FM.

Although vulvodynia isn't listed in most FM literature as one of the primary symptoms of FM, many women who have fibromyalgia also experience vulvodynia. Dr. Kim Dupree-Jones, of Oregon Health & Science University, points out that FM involves a "hypersensitivity or amplification of the central nervous system," which places the FM patient at "increased risk for any other chronic-pain condition—even localized pain such as vulvodynia." She likens the pain response in fibromyalgia to the brain being on "overdrive."

Trigger points, which are extremely sore places in the muscles (but not the same as fibromyalgia's tender points), may be the cause of vaginal pain. A myotherapist can help locate them and stretch them. *Myotherapy* is a noninvasive treatment involving the application of pressure to trigger points. A physical therapist may be able to refer you to a good myotherapist in your area. For more information on myotherapy, see Bonnie Prudden's book, *Myotherapy: A Complete Guide to Pain-Free Living*.

If you want to go the self-help route, there are exercises you can do to relieve pain in the vaginal muscles. Below, Patricia S. shares her experience with vulvodynia and how it has affected her sex life, and also describes how she has found relief both with the help of a specialist and via self-administered trigger-point therapy.

Patricia S. The vulvodynia eclipses the FM in terms of its implications for me as a woman. FM affects my life as a human being, in that it limits my energy and my ability to engage in an active lifestyle (which I used to have), and it affects my ability to eat the many foods that increase my pain. My career as a doctor gave me a definition of who I am, partly. I no longer have that. I no longer enjoy the interactions with the wide variety of people that I had at work. My life is limited to people I already know. When I meet new people, I keep my health issues to myself, which limits my talking about myself. Thank God for politics and current events—one can always talk about those topics.

Vulvodynia is a very general term. The vulva encompasses all the external portions of the female genitalia. It includes the clitoris, labia majora, labia minora, and the skin around the area. *Dynia* is Greek for "pain." Therefore, vulvodynia simply means pain in the vulval area. It causes different kinds of pain in different people. Some describe it as a rawness, burning, or aching, or a deep stabbing pain that starts in the vulva and shoots up to other places. Some people only experience the pain during intercourse; some people suffer constant burning; some people have periods of time when they are somewhat pain-free and other times when the pain worsens or is exacerbated.

Vulvodynia has taken away my ability to engage in intercourse without pain. It is too painful for me to be touched. This is a terrible loss for me. I have cut the bottom half of my body out of my life as a source of any positive activity. I think of myself as a patient in need of constant care. This has had the effect of making me feel less pretty and less desirable, with a lower self-esteem and a complete loss of libido, which I desperately want back. Before, I certainly did not value myself based on my genitals, but now I feel devastated and broken. I know that sexual relations do not have to be limited to the genitals, but nevertheless it is a tremendous loss. In addition, it is a source of conflict between me and the man in my life. He is healthy, with a normal sexual appetite, and we are unable to resolve this. The pain of the loss flares up enormously and leads to sorrow for both of us. We don't like the choices left to us, as we care very deeply for each other.

It's been hell. It was really bad. So many times, he was ready to leave me, even though we love each other. As much as I thought it would be the world's worst thing if he left me because I assumed I would never have another relationship, there were times when I just wanted to throw in the towel and say, "I can't take the tension here. I'd rather be alone." Every day there was so much screaming, crying, leaving, and agony, including his agony about not having sex. I couldn't listen to it anymore. So I started therapy to deal with the whole issue of what I've given up in life and in my relationship.

The vulvodynia has gotten better recently. I am able to have two minutes of sex once a week. In between that, we make love in other ways. It does get pretty boring for me because I can't touch my genitals with my hands, but at the same time I no longer see my vagina as something that brings pleasure. I miss the memory of being young and wanting sex on a day-to-day basis, but I have no interest in it.

I did biofeedback for a year, and it didn't help with the vulvodynia. Neither did physical therapy. Then I found a myotherapist in Florida, and I started on a regimen of pelvic-floor work. This time I found somebody who really went into the vagina and worked to release the muscles there and in the rectum. That's what she does for an hour. She puts her finger in there and works on the muscles, pressing the trigger points. There are a lot of trigger points in the vagina. Later, I figured out what she was doing, and I did it myself twice a day for a year. It's relieving some of the pain. How do I do it? I stick my thumb inside the vagina, I sit on the toilet, I pull the TV over to watch it while I work for an hour, and I press on the muscles to relieve the contractions. When you press on a muscle for a long period of time, it relaxes, and it feels so much better when it's relaxed. This therapy accomplishes myofascial release of the pelvic-floor muscles, which are inside the vagina and rectum. Doing these exercises means you learn the vagina. When you go in there all the time, you begin to recognize the muscles. Look at an anatomy book for help.

THYROID PROBLEMS

If you have FM, it's a good idea to have your thyroid gland checked out, as many women with fibromyalgia are also found to have dysfunctional thyroid glands. Checking the thyroid involves a simple blood test.

Hypothyroidism (an underactive thyroid gland) seems to be inherited. It is very common among women. Several women in my family have it. Many women benefit from medication for hypothyroidism. If you have gained weight since your diagnosis with FM, tend to be constipated, have heavy periods, or have dry skin and hair, you may need to have a low dose of thyroid hormone added to your other medications.

Over time, my thyroid gland was being destroyed by the lymphocytes and antibodies in my blood, an autoimmune condition known as *Hashimoto's thyroiditis*, which is the most common cause of hypothyroidism. The gland would have finally stopped working altogether when all the tissue was destroyed. Luckily, my rheumatologist regularly refers his patients to an endocrinologist, who diagnosed my thyroid problem and prescribed Levoxyl, which I have been taking for about five years. For the first six months, the endocrinologist adjusted the dose upward until I began to feel like I had a bit more energy and I began to lose weight. It took about a year to find the right dosage. During the first seven years of my diagnosis, I'd put on about forty pounds, and in the last several years I have lost thirty-five of those pounds. I believe my thyroid hormones are finally regulated. I take 125 mcg (micrograms) of Levoxyl in the morning. I also take 50 mg (milligrams) of the supplement DHEA and one tablet of Drenamin. Drenamin is made of dried bovine adrenal gland. It helps the adrenal gland return to normal functioning. I seem to have more energy when I regularly take these two supplements.

> **Val T.** I have hypothyroidism (Hashimoto's), which cropped up less than a year ago. I was fatigued, had night sweats, panic attacks, increased pain, weight gain, sluggishness, and insomnia. The insomnia prohibited the deepest, most important sleep stage, delta sleep, when we heal and produce hormones. It is the restorative sleep most people take for granted. With FM, it is difficult to achieve delta sleep without meds. So for people with FM, a small injury is compounded because they lack the hormones to heal. The lack of delta sleep increased all my pain levels.
>
> My hypothyroidism also caused sensitivity to cold, or Raynaud's disease, as well as changes in my skin and hair. It greatly affected my FM, due to the overlapping symptoms. I have noticed that many people who have FM also have thyroid problems.
>
> I didn't notice a difference in my FM when I started taking Synthroid (thyroid hormone). Now when I forget to take it, I notice that I suffer more fatigue than usual.

HORMONE REPLACEMENT THERAPY

When we women reach our mid- to late thirties, our levels of estrogen and progesterone drop, and we experience changes in our body, libido, mood, and sleep habits. These conditions can aggravate FM symptoms, and vice versa. An imbalance in one's hormones may also intensify PMS, menstrual, and perimeno-pausal difficulties, as well as promote osteoporosis.

Hormone replacement therapy (HRT) is an option to keep in mind. However, recent results from an ongoing study called the Women's Health Initiative showed a higher incidence of heart disease in women undergoing HRT, which has raised concerns about HRT's safety. One discussion of the study pointed out that although the number of women on HRT who contracted heart disease (164 women out of 8,506 on HRT) was considered statistically significant when compared to the number of women on placebo who contracted heart disease (29 percent more than the 122 women taking placebo who contracted heart disease), the actual number was also small enough to be considered "slight" (164 out of 8,506 women equals 1.92 percent). Additionally, the data measuring quality of life from the same study (energy level, sexual desire, skin and hair quality, etc.) have not yet been analyzed. It should also be pointed out that this study involved a particular combination of hormones. There are several different types of HRT available, including both natural and synthetic forms of hormones. As with any treatment, it's up to you to decide what is best for your body.

> **Diane H.** I've been postmenopausal since age forty-nine. Since using progesterone cream and being off estrogen for a year and a half, I've been doing fine hormonally. Most importantly, the depression has resolved, so I no longer take antidepressants.

▲▲▲

One of the frustrating aspects of living with fibromyalgia is that it tends to confuse other health matters that may or may not be related to FM. This seems especially true when we start discussing hormonal issues, as Victoria's story shows:

> **Victoria M.** I remember saying to my gynecologist about fifteen years ago that when I ovulated I felt like I was going to lose the lot, because the incredible weight in my lower abdomen felt as though it was about to respond to gravity. His response: "I hope you

don't." I also grew little black hairs on my chin. He maintained that I had a hormonal imbalance, but in his words, "Hormonal imbalances are more difficult to correct than they are to live with." He obviously was not the one who had to live with it! My menstrual cycles were regular in terms of the calendar, but I was very mindful of my strained back and the general aches in my legs, all of which would abate after the onset of menstruation. My period was very heavy and of long duration. My endeavors to find the cause and effect for these problems were fruitless, so I managed the best way I could. A naturopath I consulted with several years ago declared I had hormonal imbalances. I was only forty-one at the time, and I laughingly remarked that I was too young for menopause. His response to my comment was, "I am not referring to menopause." That left me thinking about what sort of hormones he was talking about.

So it is not just the illness and the interaction of each of these conditions that make life with FM very difficult to manage, but the clearly unfortunate, unwarranted, additional "diagnoses" from the uneducated.

Rae H. In 1982, I had a total hysterectomy due to endometriosis, and I began hormone replacement therapy immediately. Over the years, we had an increasingly difficult time controlling the hot flashes. I've often wondered if the hot flashes might have been complicated by the FM.

Patricia S. I wasn't menopausal when I got FM and vulvodynia at age forty-three. (I've since gone through menopause in the last couple years.) At the time, I was not using hormones even though I was in a perimenopausal state, because who'd heard of perimenopause nine years ago? I didn't know my hormones were beginning to wind down, because I was getting my periods regularly. Who thinks about their hormone levels when they're getting their period every month? Eventually my doctors put me on hormone therapy, but it never helped. It did nothing. Even though I thought I was taking a good dose, I wasn't getting enough. I was using vaginal hormones twice a day and oral hormones twice a day. Still, it was as if I were doing nothing.

Then I found a physician in Phoenix who is a vulva specialist. There are a number of such specialists, but I trust him the most.

He's the best. He informed me that my vagina was atrophied from all the hormones I was taking. Inside my vagina, where I can't see, the flesh was very thin and red. I couldn't believe that all the gynecologists who had examined me for my problems with vaginal infection had never told me that. (Somehow the environment in my vagina had become deranged and open to infection, so I'd been to a few gynecologists over the years to deal with the resulting bacterial and yeast infections.) When my new doctor informed me of the state of my vagina, I said, "Really? Nobody's ever told me that." He put me on a very high dose of hormones. He went really mainstream, prescribing Cenestin, which is a drug-company conjugated estrogen. I don't really like the idea of using that kind of product, but I went along with his game. And I grew my vagina back.

GAINING NEW PERSPECTIVES

A recurring theme in many women's comments to me is how living with FM has forced them to reexamine their place in the world as women. This can mean many things: finding new ways to feel beautiful, placing less value on doing and more on being, redefining your roles at home and at work. Many times, it means tapping into previously untested strengths.

Cybill C. I have learned so much as a woman. I've learned to appreciate the good days much more. And I've learned that I can have chronic illness and still be sexy and funny.

Sisu G. I've learned that it's just as stupid to try to be a socially appropriate woman when I have FM as it was when I was normal. In fact, I've seen it demonstrated that not wearing makeup does not make the monster police come and take me away. Do I try to shave my legs and be pretty anyway? Well, yes. And I still like dressing up. But now I view it less as something I have to do, and I worry less about being a cookie-cutter model. I see how much energy some women waste trying to look like each other, and I think how wonderful the world could be if they turned that energy toward issues like getting equal pay for equal work, or like recycling. The energy that goes into the ideal of the cookie-cutter model is immense, and most people never have anything to measure it against. Dealing with this illness has given me a new perspective.

Val T. I'm still "Mom!" I just don't do as much maintenance on the house as before. Now I concentrate on my family and on making them happy and doing nice things for them. I have a lot more time for them now than I did before, which is what life and love should be about. Housework and my job are not so important anymore. My family and their needs come first.

Before I met my doctor, I underwent a huge change in my role as a mother and wife. A lot of things were put on hold when I was very ill, and I felt like I was losing everything that was important to me. I have been very fortunate to have had many understanding doctors who believed in me.

Katie G. As a woman, I have been pleased to discover my ability to comfort and nurture myself. I know what to do and not do. I've realized how strong—emotionally, spiritually, mentally, and physically—I am and that I am a survivor. I've discovered that I possess a lot of tenacity and endurance for the long haul.

Taking Care of Ourselves: Treatment Options for Fibromyalgia

What do you as a unique woman with fibromyalgia need to do to take care of yourself? What is the right treatment approach for you in particular? Once the diagnosis of FM is established, you and your doctors can start to determine the answers to these questions. Discuss each of your symptoms with your health-care providers and decide on a way to begin. What symptoms are bothering you the most? (Usually sleep difficulties and pain are reported at the top of the list.) Should you use medications? Supplements? Herbs, homeopathic remedies, or a combination of the two? What type of exercise or physical therapy should you try? Each of these treatments can help. However, every patient with FM is different, and not all medications and treatments bring the same relief. Even if you embark on a path of treatment that ultimately proves unhelpful, don't get discouraged. Keep trying until you find the right combination of therapies that works for you.

In this chapter, our survey respondents write about the many and varied ways they care for themselves as women living with fibromyalgia. The goals of reducing pain and fatigue through the use of remedies ranging from regular exercise to movement therapies, from conventional medications to alternative treatments, are among the subjects discussed. But first, let's establish what the most important tool is for taking care of yourself.

SELF-CARE STARTS WITH OURSELVES

Fibromyalgia is a complex syndrome. Having a solid foundation of care providers who understand the illness and are willing to partner with you in your health care is half the battle. Your involvement is the other very important half. No one knows how you feel but you, and you are your best advocate. Ultimately, the choice of treatment plan is up to you.

Sondra H.   First and foremost, I rely on myself for my primary care. I am the one who feels and deals with this, day in and day out, so I must take a proactive role in my health-care management. My primary-care physician is there to help, and I see my rheumatologist twice a year. My time at the pain clinic taught me how to manage my health so that I'm not constantly in the doctors' offices. They are there when I need them, but there's only so much they can do. The rest is up to each one of us, individually.

Patricia S.   My primary-care person is myself. No one is ever going to be as good an advocate for you as yourself. No one is ever going to know you so well. No doctor has the time. No doctor can ever understand the whole picture, as they are not inside you, feeling what you feel. They understand only what they want to with all their own biases. (It's like the old cliché of the elephant and six blind men. The man touching the elephant's trunk believes the creature most resembles a snake; the one touching its side maintains it is very like a wall; the one holding the tail believes it must be a rope; each of them is convinced his perspective is the "right" one.) Doctors only know an "average" of all patients, not the individual. And very often a person does not fit the textbook description. No one is ever as clear as the textbook. We all have our own chemistries, yet few doctors avoid a one-size-fits-all attitude. I go to specialists based on what part of the puzzle I think they can help with. I must coordinate my care, as it is multidimensional. I trust no one. When I've tried to expand my caretakers' knowledge, I've met with, at best, a benign indifference to what the other caretaker has done or, at worst, an opinion that what the other is doing is foolish.

Donna F.   Taking care of myself becomes an all-day, everyday project. It involves many kinds of fulfilling activities, including spiritual (prayer, reading), physical (exercise, appearance, diet), medical, mental, and emotional. In all, on a good day I might spend approximately four to five hours trying to take proper care of myself. On a bad day, I'm down all day, feeling like my body is in great need of rest and repair. For the most part my days are a combination of good times, used to accomplish goals, and bad times, used to rest and reenergize.

Diane H.   In the past five years, I have eliminated my prolonged bouts with chronic fatigue and reduced my bodily pain to a manageable level with fewer flare-ups. I have done this through the following "treatments":

1.   Maintaining a positive attitude and outlook. I think FM involves a genetic predisposition and that my lifestyle— my eating, drinking, and smoking habits—eventually brought it into being. I think of FM as "God's way of making me slow down." I deal with it. I don't focus on what I can't do. I focus on what I can still do;

2.   Massage therapy once a month (more often during flare-ups);

3.   Avoiding alcohol, diet sodas, chocolate, fried foods, red meat, fast foods, and prepackaged foods;

4.   Exercise—even walking and mild weight training—two to five days a week;

5.   Water exercise during the summer (our local pool is outdoors, and isn't kept warm enough to use during the winter months).

Initially, taking care of myself required most of the day. I would go to either aquatic therapy, massage therapy, or an exercise class; commuting, dressing, changing, etc., took about two hours. I needed intermittent rest periods of twenty minutes to half an hour.

Pain flare-ups required alternating ice and heat packs or a hot bath or time in the Jacuzzi, which took another hour or two. Now that I'm feeling better, my treatment plan includes a daily walk, massage therapy once a month, and basically listening to my body. If I'm tired or feeling poorly, I take it easy. If I'm feeling good, the challenge is to avoid overdoing.

I took a medical leave of absence from work right after my FM diagnosis and began reading all I could about the illness. When immediate relief was not in sight, and after suffering almost a year with various symptoms, I quit my job and increased my relaxation, traveling, healthier eating, and walking program, despite my pain and lack of energy. In early 1997, I consulted a naturopathic physician and focused on nutrition; I also joined Weight Watchers. In addition, I consulted a physician outside my insurance coverage for possible thyroid problems. He diagnosed Wilson's syndrome (low T3 thyroid hormone) and prescribed 25 mcg (micrograms) of Cytomel, which "cured" my chronic fatigue within three days! Up to that point, the pain had been manageable, but the fatigue had been crippling.

▲▲▲

Note that the common theme throughout these women's comments is that they have been the ones to coordinate all the different facets of their treatment, rather than waiting for someone else to tell them what steps to take next. Research proves that people with a potentially terminal illness have a higher survival rate if they take a proactive role in managing their health care. Although FM isn't deadly, a similar principle seems to apply: Patients who stay proactively involved in their self-care enjoy better success in reducing their symptoms and creating a higher quality of life.

EXERCISE

Specialists in FM recommend a regular program of gentle exercise. Even though exercising may at first increase your pain, sticking with it often greatly improves symptoms, as my own experience attests. I was very active before FM, but I didn't walk regularly or do any aerobic exercise. Since my diagnosis, I have discovered that regular exercise is one of the most effective treatments for FM pain. Exercise helps reduce pain by loosening my tight muscles. It is also beneficial for my anxiety, depression, and digestion. It's a great stress reducer. It has even helped with the pain of my regular headaches. I also know that I am at less risk for injury when I exercise regularly.

I was sent to physical therapy right after diagnosis. It helped to set the proactive tone for my FM self-care program. The exercises my physical therapist taught me have proved invaluable. One of the best lessons I learned in PT is to sit up straight in a chair and to use a back cushion. Before FM, I would lie on the sofa and watch a video or read—or worse yet, lie in bed and read. I have broken that lifelong habit and now use either a straight-backed chair or an old wooden rocker that has ergonomic cushions for my back and allows me to place my feet flat on the floor. This has helped both my headaches and my lower-back problems.

I'm not alone in finding benefit from exercise. Other FM'ers extol the advantages of such low-impact activities as walking, swimming, water aerobics, bike riding, stretching/yoga, and tai chi. Whatever activity you choose, be creative with your exercise program! Below, Linda M. describes the role belly dance plays in her life with fibromyalgia. Choosing an exercise you love to do, as Linda has, makes it fun and something to look forward to. In addition, it adds another important facet to your self-care program: regular participation in activities you enjoy and find fulfilling.

There are many types of exercise programs available. To locate a pool or an exercise class for people with chronic pain, contact your local YMCA or a nearby chapter of the Arthritis Foundation. As another option, water aerobics for seniors is often a great option for FM patients. And the book *Get Fit While You Sit: Easy Workouts from Your Chair*, by Charlene Torkelson, outlines exercise programs for those with health or movement restrictions (see Resources). Consider combining regular walking with a movement system such as the Feldenkrais Method (described in this chapter) or the Alexander Technique. Or try a mixture of yoga and water aerobics. Success seems to come to exercisers who *like* their workouts. They have fun and don't look at exercise simply as one more task to speed through.

When choosing a physical therapist or trainer, ask them if they are well acquainted with FM. If not, find one who is, if possible. Using the right technique and pacing yourself is so important, and a professional familiar with this condition can guide you appropriately. Whether you exercise with the help of a specialist or on your own, start slowly, and see how you feel a day or two later. If your activity causes you to experience added pain and fatigue, rest and back off a little. Only increase the intensity or duration of your exercise if it helps you feel better—that is, less stiff and sore. Remember, we don't always feel the effects of an activity right away; with FM, pain and stiffness might not hit until a few days after the activity. Hold back and make sure the exercise you have chosen is the right one for you. There is a delicate balance between exercising for pain relief and better cardiovascular health and exercising your way to a flare-up.

Finally, stretching is very important to include in any exercise program, and it is imperative for FM patients. In addition to stretching as a part of your exercise routine, it is also beneficial to stretch during regular daily activities, such as after periods of sitting or standing.

The bottom line is this: Choose an exercise program and keep moving.

Gerry L. Finally, after years of trying to exercise, I am having success with it. But only because I am being consistent and taking it slowly. Progress, not perfection. If all I can do is get in the warm water or whirlpool, that is doing something. After all, I could just stay home and feel sorry for myself. On other days I do my warm-water physical-therapy routine and use an underwater treadmill. I feel so good. I'm doing something for my whole self.

Suzan B. For many of the first years of my illness, I could not even walk down the block. I slowly worked up to walking one house down and back, until now I can go for a walk. At this point, I can keep myself from being bedridden by walking once a week. If I do not walk, I will quickly deteriorate until I cannot walk and cannot do anything else to take care of myself, even basic self-care.

Walking helps my neurological symptoms. It keeps me out of depression, and it keeps me warmer, of all the silly things. Before I was able to walk, I was cold all the time. As long as I keep walking, I stay warmer. The improved circulation also helps my immune system by emptying my glands. I have to drink massive amounts of water in order to walk, which brings its own benefits. Walking also helps my body's oxygenation processes. I just learned that people with chronic fatigue and immune dysfunction syndrome (CFIDS) and FM absorb oxygen as poorly as someone with congestive heart failure. Heavy breathing, promoted by walking, helps.

Donna P. During the early stages of my fibromyalgia, the doctor had me doing water therapy. It seemed to be the best form of exercise for me, but I could not afford to go since my insurance refused to pay for it. In its place, walking seems to work best. Sometimes I can walk a long time and other times only for ten minutes.

Linda M. FM patients are often advised to swim for exercise. I don't like to swim, but I love the art of Middle Eastern belly dance. So I was pleased to learn from a psychiatrist that belly dancing is similar to swimming! Like moving in the water, belly dance creates a gentle resistance to muscles. When you belly dance, you aren't jarring your joints the way you would if you were doing aerobic exercise.

Before the car accident that led to my FM, I had studied belly dance for ten years. For the first few years after the accident, when my pain was all-consuming, I didn't miss dancing much. But as time went on, I began to long for the joy it brought me, the exercise I needed, and the physical and mental release of being transported into a world where pain did not exist.

I was talking about it on the telephone with my mother when she lamented, "Oh, Linda, you'll never dance again!"

At first, I was crushed. Then my old spirit rose along with the hairs on the back of my neck.

"Oh yes I will!" I said. And right then I decided to accept the fact that my pain wasn't going away and that I would dance anyway. Years later, Mom was embarrassed to have said what she did, but in retrospect I'm grateful for her "shock therapy." It was the catalyst I needed to start taking charge of my life again.

I signed up once again for belly-dance lessons, and after a few years I began performing occasionally in restaurants. In 1999, a persistent friend persuaded me to teach belly-dance classes. (Although I was able to start dancing again before I found a physician who was willing to help me manage pain, I couldn't teach dance without pain management.)

I find teaching to be tremendously rewarding and satisfying. When I look at my students standing behind me in the mirror during class, I see smiling faces, women who are trimming inches as their bodies become more toned and graceful. And I think, "I gave them these gifts!"

If I'm feeling tired before class, dancing gives me energy. I have actually extended classes by as much as half an hour, because I get so involved I don't realize how late it is until someone has to leave!

Belly dance is more than a beautiful distraction from pain. In addition to the physical exercise provided by the dancing, listening to music causes our bodies to release endorphins, our own natural painkillers. Some hospitals use music in conjunction with pain medications to lessen pain. And there's nothing like wearing chiffon, sequins, and sparkles to boost your spirits when your symptoms are making you feel like last year's faded rosebush.

I've learned to prepare my students in advance so they won't be shocked or worried when one of my FM symptoms appear. At the beginning of each new session, I inform my students that I have fibromyalgia and give them a brief explanation of the symptoms that can affect my dance. Sometimes my balance is off, so if I seem a little tippy when I demonstrate a move, I am! And since I stiffen up after I've been sitting cross-legged for a while, I'll hobble around for a minute when I stand up again. There will be times when I won't be able to remember a student's name or a particular word because my short-term memory is affected. And I've learned from experience just how many repetitions of a particular warm-up exercise I can do without hurting myself, so I'm not cheating when I stop doing repetitions but ask my students to continue.

It helps to have a sense of humor. I tell my dance students, "Now that I have fibromyalgia, I can't perform a back bend—but then I couldn't do a back bend before I had fibromyalgia, either!"

Rachel B. I like to do outdoor activities/sports, physically pushing my strength to the limit. When I don't feel too good, I resort to cross-stitching, whenever my eyes and concentration let me. At times, doing the household chores is physically challenging enough, and I need frequent rest periods.

Diane H. I have been "exercise intolerant" for most of my life, and I don't really understand why. Two doctors suggested it's because of my mitral-valve prolapse syndrome. Two suggested it's because of my fibromyalgia. The cardiologist said it could be either. I started a walking program in 1986, walking one to three miles, three to six mornings a week, and I quit smoking in 1987, and yet today I still can't walk up a short flight of stairs or any kind of incline without getting winded. I've also included weight and resistance training at our fitness center since November 1999, which has increased my strength and ability to lift, reach, and do more household chores, even though it also increases my heart rate more rapidly than I think it should.

I've done aquatic therapy with a certified Arthritis Foundation aquatic therapist, and it was wonderful. (I left the program when we moved to southern Arizona.) It relieves stress and makes exercising easier. Where I live now, during the summer I go to the outdoor pool for water aerobics.

I'm no longer able to play weekly golf—heck, I'm not able to play golf at all most of the time! If I play nine holes when I'm not hurting, afterward I'm totally exhausted and can't move. I go to bed and sleep for ten to twelve hours, and the next day I feel like a Mack truck has run over me.

I haven't been able to do any hiking. I can walk two to three miles on level surfaces, but any inclines totally wipe me out. When we travel and there's a hike to somewhere special (like Cape Flattery on the Olympic Peninsula or to a waterfall), it takes me twice as long as a normal person to reach the destination, and I have to allow that I'll pretty much be wiped out the next day.

Emma L. Recently I started to swim again, which requires I be at the pool at one P.M. for the inexpensive senior-hour swim. Fortunately, the pool is very close to where I live.

Sisu G. I take tai chi classes three days a week. I tried physical therapy, but the therapist wasn't used to dealing with a patient who is already doing stretches and strength-building exercises, so she put me on an exercise bike, tiring me out and doing more harm than good. I own an exercise bike; I could do that at home if I had the energy. So I don't go to her anymore. I'll be finding a new therapist. My doctor recommended tai chi. It has helped me build up strength in my skeletal muscle structure where it is doing me the most good. I have a greater pain tolerance, and the amount of listening to my body involved (it's important to choose a class with a good balance between strength and stillness) has actually helped me change how my body responds to sensation. Some of what used to be pain is now only sensation. It doesn't take care of all the pain, but I no longer feel as overcome by it as I used to.

   The tai chi class is painful. We do half an hour of stretching and half an hour of tai chi and then sometimes a lot of push-ups and so on afterwards. I can do about twenty crunches and about ten push-ups. I can't do any after it starts to burn—that's when it will really do me damage if I continue. I'm not to expend 100 percent energy on anything, ever, if I can help it. To do so will cause even more pain.

   I can't run or jump around much; I have about three minutes of energy before high-aerobic exercises start to burn. My doctors don't know why this is. But if I don't pay attention to it, I'll be in a world of bigger hurt for days afterwards. I do low-impact, moderate exercise as often as I can. I have to rest between activities. I get to tai chi an hour early and sit down, maybe stretch my legs a little, but mostly I sit till it's time for class. It's like having a bad rechargeable battery—I recharge, but not completely. If I rest, I will be able to do more, but I'll run out of energy fast if I keep going back to do more again and again.

   Most of my tai chi classmates understand about my illness. My rule is that I go no matter how I feel, and I don't cry during class. I frequently cry afterwards, because it hurts. My doctors were very up-front about this. They told me that it would hurt so much that I would wish they'd put a morphine lick in the gym. They were right; it does. And I do. But I go, and I participate.

▲▲▲

MOVEMENT THERAPIES: SOMATICS AND FELDENKRAIS

I have included in this chapter the comments of two practitioners of movement therapies: Ed Barrera, who teaches a technique known as somatics, and Jane McClenney, a Certified Feldenkrais Practitioner. Both of these exercise systems have helped me in my efforts to take care of myself.

Somatics

Ed Barrera is an FM'er who used exercise to get on the road to recovery. For four years I have used the Muscle Balance and Function (MBF) program he taught me. I try to do the exercises every night, even when I am exhausted. When I began the program I noticed an immediate difference in how I felt. My weight was balanced during standing, my muscles seemed looser, and I was building muscle for the first time. Ed asked me to pay attention to how I use my right side, the side that is always in pain. For example, I learned that I approached the light switch or the sink or the door from my right side, not straight on. I was overusing some muscles, while not using others at all. Now I also use somatics along with MBF. Over the years I have used MBF and now somatics exercises to relax myself. I feel calm and peaceful afterward. For me, these exercise systems have continued to improve the pain of FM.

What Is Somatics? How Does It Help a Female FM Client? How Has It Helped Me?

by Ed Barrera

Hanna Somatic Education is a form of body work and movement practice that frees the body of its neuromuscular contractions and compensated postures. The typical session consists of hands-on body work with a certified Hanna Somatic Educator to reeducate various parts of the body about its movement potential. The work is very gentle; its aim is to free the muscles' and joints' abilities to move more easily and naturally, thereby reducing the contracted state of the muscles. As a client learns to become more aware of the internal sensations of this movement education, she will typically sense the effects of releasing formerly contracted, sore, painful areas.

The client is also instructed in a few simple home-care movements. All the movements are easy-to-do, gentle, nonexercise types of movement that remind the central nervous system (CNS) to "pay attention to" a particular muscle group or area. The movements are designed to be accomplished with the least effort possible. Special attention is given so a client learns how to move more easily and well within her ability to do so. The client feels and senses the release of tension in the targeted area.

Traditionally, many people are taught to stretch a muscle. During conventional stretching activities, at a neurological level, a message is sent by the brain to the various muscles involved, and that muscle area will contract and say, "Okay, that's the limit." So you may try for months or years to "stretch" your muscles with no apparent gain. In fact, if you try to overexert, your muscles will further contract, setting off this reflex. If, by contrast, you were to learn how to contract a specific muscle area, then the CNS will "pay attention" and will allow the lengthening of the targeted area. The result will be fully felt and you will sense a relaxation, among other sensations, thus freeing up the area. Eventually the client is taught a ten-minute program which, if practiced, will allow the neuromuscular system to remain supple, graceful, coordinated, balanced, and pain free.

Typically, my female FM clients have postures that exhibit misalignment and compensated motion so that their muscles are chronically contracted, painful to move, sensitive to touch, and generally always "on." The CNS continues over time to send messages that keep the various muscles in habitually contracted states. Thomas Hanna, the founder of the somatics movement program, called this mechanism *sensory motor amnesia* and defined it as places in the body where one cannot sense or feel how the muscles are supposed to contract and then release in a more balanced way. The result of this is movements that are stiff, unbalanced, difficult, and painful.

With FM, even while you sleep, the CNS keeps sending these distorted messages to the muscles, so that when you awake your muscles are still contracted, you are still achy and stiff, and it's another day of pain. Then because of the lack of restorative sleep, your muscles have to work that much harder when you need them, and you lack the energy you once had. It is because of the messages from the nervous system that the muscles contract in various states and places and you become "practiced" at fatigue. Of course, our stressful daily lives impact this vicious cycle.

With the Hanna Somatic Education process you learn how to voluntarily contract an area and then how to lengthen it; you learn how to keep the musculoskeletal system in better balance. This allows you to feel more relaxed and experience less "brain fog," because your mind and body are now more balanced. You will notice an increase in vitality, energy, and freedom to move naturally, which translates to a life with less pain.

For myself, a former FM'er, my ability to accomplish daily activities is increasingly improving, whether it's carrying the groceries, washing the dishes, or cleaning the car. All of these formerly painful activities are now a joy. In fact, my activity level is now at a point where I ski, play soccer, ride a bike, etc., all without pain and muscle soreness the following day—unless of course I fall, which happens with skiing and playing soccer. I'm also an instructor of a yoga-based movement program, and even those movements have become easier and more effortless. In any event, now I have a tool that helps me almost instantly recover from the trauma of these events and of life's daily stresses—if I practice my daily movement program. And the movements themselves are a pleasure; I could not imagine any other activity that is so easy to accomplish and that allows me to go on with life, and even to improve over time.

Eduardo Barrera is a Somatic Educator in the tradition of Thomas Hanna and a nationally certified Resistance Training Specialist (RTS1). Audiocassettes of his program are available from Gravity Werks (see Resources).

The Feldenkrais Method

Moshe Feldenkrais (1904–1984) began developing the techniques that eventually became the Feldenkrais Method in the late 1940s. He was born in the Ukraine and later moved to Paris, where he earned a degree in mechanical engineering and a Ph.D. in physics. He worked in the nuclear-research lab with Fredric Joliot-Curie. He was the first European to earn a black belt in judo and was largely responsible for bringing judo to Western culture. After suffering a crippling knee injury playing soccer, Feldenkrais taught himself to walk again without pain or reinjury. Over a period of years he explored how to teach others what he'd learned. Later he developed these movements into two systems: Awareness Through Movement and Functional Integration, collectively known as the Feldenkrais Method.

The Feldenkrais Method is a gentle, commonsense, educational approach that teaches people how to improve their movement. In group or individual lessons with a practitioner, people learn to develop easier, more efficient, more comfortable movement, thus easing pain and improving posture and balance, even with an infirmity, disability, or illness.

Since most of us don't think about how we move until we experience pain, limitation, or injury, we end up moving in habitual, automatic, and inefficient ways for a long time before we do anything about it. Unfortunately, these habitual movements are usually those we perform repeatedly at our jobs, sports, and hobbies, which makes everyday life less than ideal.

The Feldenkrais Method enables people to become more aware of how they move themselves in their environment; it teaches them to move efficiently and easily, reducing stress on their body so a problem or pain does not continue.

Feldenkrais involves two different kinds of lessons: Awareness Through Movement (ATM) and Functional Integration (FI). In Awareness Through Movement, the teacher verbally directs students through a sequence of movements that enable them to shift out of old habits, discovering new possibilities of moving. Lessons are forty-five minutes to an hour in duration, and students lie on the floor on mats, stand, or sit in chairs. Students begin noticing changes as movement becomes more pleasurable, even with the first lesson.

In Functional Integration, practitioners work one-on-one with a student for about an hour, guiding them with slow, gentle touch. These movements send new information directly to the neuro-muscular system, helping the student to develop more efficient movement with less effort. FI is custom tailored to the specific needs of the student.

Jane McClenney, Certified Feldenkrais Practitioner, writes:

I both teach the Awareness Through Movement classes and work individually with clients. I work with many people with neurological disorders, chronic pain problems, injuries, and muscle disorders. A number of my students have fibromyalgia, and they get relief from taking the weekly class. Students relax in a very deep way during class and get in touch with the patterns of holding that they have developed with fibromyalgia. We all "guard" against pain, and I find that most people with fibromyalgia in particular hold musculature in their rib cage very tightly. When they are able to find ways to let this go to some extent, their breathing improves, as does their ability to move with more freedom and less chronic pain. During a class I observe where a student is experiencing difficulties moving, and in subsequent classes I plan a lesson that speaks to their particular area of difficulty.

When Mari Skelly first came to my class, she endured a great deal of pain in her rib cage and shoulders. After a series of classes she was amazed at how much more easily she could move and at how the constant pain in her rib cage was relieved. She was able to breathe more fully and thereby improve her comfort level. Because Feldenkrais is an educational model, she has learned additional skills to help herself by using Feldenkrais when she does experience pain. For fibromyalgia patients, Feldenkrais provides an experience of being in more control of their pain and their ability to function. They gain skills to help themselves maintain more freedom of movement, as well as skills that aid them in their self-care.

MEDICATIONS

This section aims to give you a good idea of the variety of medications women use for FM. The classes of pharmaceuticals typically used to treat FM include antidepressants, pain medications, sleep aids, and muscle relaxants. Many kinds of each of these are available through your doctor. (Also see Chapter 12 for a discussion of new drug-treatment approaches for FM.)

The goal of treating FM with pharmaceuticals is to find a drug or combination of drugs that alleviates your symptoms enough to allow you to participate in life. When you are in constant pain, it's hard to concentrate and all your energy is required just to get through the day. Work with your doctor to find the medications that allow you to do more. You want to be able to exercise, work around the house, and concentrate on your life, not your pain.

It takes time and patience to find the medications and dosages that will help your pain and fatigue. The majority of women who took part in the survey for this book tried a variety of medications until they found a combination that worked well for them. Most FM patients have told me that finding the right drug not only took time but also that the dosage had to be adjusted and readjusted to determine the exact amount that helped them with their symptoms but didn't bombard their bodies with side effects. Many women with FM take only small dosages of medications, as our systems are sensitive to start with. Trying a small dose of any new medication is always a good way to begin.

Here are a few important points to remember when working with your doctor to find the right medications:

◀ Don't give up until you have the right combination. This means being up-front with your doctor about side effects, rather than just enduring them or discontinuing use of the drug without informing your doctor. Often, a side effect such as constipation can be dealt with easily and the medication can be continued. It's very important to mention any side effect, no matter how small. Then your doctor can decide whether it's best to try another drug or to work on the side effects first;

◄ Most importantly, tell your doctor about any other medications you are currently using, including any over-the-counter drugs or supplements. Your doctor and pharmacist can make sure all your medications are compatible;

◄ Remember that medication is just one part of your treatment plan. Finding the right drug protocol can allow you a measure of pain relief so that the other, equally important ways of working on your illness can be addressed.

Now hear from some of the women about their experiences with medication. *Important note*: Do not attempt to follow the treatment plans advocated by these individuals without first consulting with your doctor.

Donnie M.   One thing I have learned is that FM patients are extremely sensitive to medications and must be very careful about what they take. I never try a new medication without my husband being with me, and if possible I always try just half the tablet first. I have a lot of fear when trying something new.

Suzan B.   I have a prescription for medical marijuana, and I cannot walk without it. It lessens the severity of my symptoms the next day, although I still have some. It allows me to tolerate my FM pain, and it mitigates my neurological symptoms.

Jean T.   For quite some time my doctor was struggling with what on earth he could give me for the extreme pain I have experienced for several years. I cannot use any of the traditional pain meds. The side effects are worse than the pain. He overheard my sister say she knew several people with FM who were taking Prozac for pain. He said, "Let's try it." It works. The next day, the pain was so diminished as to be nonexistent.

I hesitate to give all the credit to the Prozac, as I also started using a microcurrent device known as the Alpha Stim, which delivers an electrical impulse that interrupts pain messages to the brain. If I am not feeling too well when I wake up (brain fog, stiffness, and extreme tiredness), I'll use the Alpha Stim for one hour, and then I am ready to face the day.

Sisu G. I take 5 mg of Flexeril (a muscle relaxant) at night for four weeks, then I reduce the dosage for three days and stop for four. This way, I don't build up too much of a tolerance. Yesterday, my doctor gave me Ultram (a nonnarcotic pain reliever) to try when I need it most on bad days. It's usually prescribed to take much more often than I do, but I don't want to be on a constant painkiller.

I've also tried antidepressants. I will be trying a low dose of Celexa for the pain and fatigue. I tried Elavil; it gave me awful nightmares and I couldn't tolerate it. I tried Zoloft and I hated it. I tolerated it pretty well but I got a sense of overstimulation. Lights and noises were too much. I had a creepy, crawling, itchy feeling to my bones, so I stopped taking any of those for about two months, and that did me a lot of good. The pain is greater, but I feel more present and more whole. The downside of using antidepressants for FM is that while they do good things for pain and fatigue, and while a good many FM patients also have depression as a symptom, not all of us do, and there's no way to eliminate the mental effects of the drugs. We'll see what happens with Celexa. If it doesn't work, I simply won't take it.

Gina H. The only things I am doing now are taking medication; seeing a psychologist, a pain doctor, and a bone doctor; and seeing a chaplain once a week. The medications I'm taking are Neurontin (for nerve-pain reduction), OxyContin (an analgesic), Xanax (an antianxiety drug), Phenergan (an antihistamine), Dyazide (a diuretic), Estrace (estrogen), Lipitor (a cholesterol reducer), Zomig (normally used to treat severe migraines), Senokot-S (a laxative), and Tylenol every day.

I've tried epidural injections, trigger-point injections, medications from A to Z, walking, aerobics, biofeedback, and meditation. I have been anointed, touched by hands, and prayed over. I have used a sauna, therapeutic massage, and healing tapes. I thought that each of these methods would work, but they didn't, so I've just given up on all of them except medication and praying.

Denise P. At bedtime I take two Vicodin 5/500 mg tabs, Vioxx 25 mg, and clonazepam 1 mg. During the day I take Sinemet 25/250 mg, one tablet four times a day; Neurontin 300 mg, one tablet four times a day; Glucophage 500 mg for diabetes, two tabs twice a day; and Ultram 50 mg as needed for pain during the day. I do water exercises and I have had physical therapy on and off over the years for pain in my neck and back.

I've only been diagnosed for about two years, so most of the medications have helped so far. At first I only took the Ultram for pain, and it worked at night. After about a year or so, I added one Vicodin at bedtime.

Emma L. I have now completely dropped antidepressants. I had taken low doses of Paxil since about 1992, when, after treatment for Graves' disease (a type of hypothyroidism), the symptoms did not go away. Paxil seemed to help with the fatigue, but I recently discovered some side effects which made me discontinue it. My Kaiser health-plan doctor did not like that. He tried me on the antidepressant trazodone (Desyrel), which I also discontinued because I did not think it helped. I take Levothroid for the thyroid. I take naproxen and ibuprofen for the muscle pains, with little results. Over-the-counter MSM (methyl sulfonyl methane, used for muscle-pain relief) seemed to help for a while. It does help over the long run if taken regularly in a dose of at least 1,500 mg per day.

I read and research a lot and try the possible alternatives I read about. The year 2001 was very rough because it was determined that I now also have osteoporosis and arthritis. I take Fosamax for the osteoporosis. Warmth helps with the muscle pain, especially moist heat. On some days Sudafed helps with fatigue. St. John's wort did not; it just made me jumpy and nervous.

Val T. I take supplements: malic acid 1,200 mg a day, magnesium 300 mg a day, grape-seed extract, flaxseed oil, vitamin E, and a multivitamin. My prescription meds include Ultram four times a day. It works great and is proven effective for FM. I also take trazodone, an antidepressant, 100–200 mg at bedtime for sleep. It helps me to achieve delta sleep. I take Zanaflex, a relatively new muscle relaxant, 1 mg four times a day. I walk every day. I stopped using the TENS unit (a device to send electrical impulses through the body, similar to the Alpha Stim) per doctor's orders. It caused scarring on my back from using it twenty-four/seven.

Donna P. I take Flexeril for the aches and pains, Serzone for depression, and amitriptyline for sleep. I used to take the sleeping pill Ambien, and it worked great, but my insurance company refused to cover it. I also was on Prilosec for my GERD (gastro-esophageal reflux disease); now I take a different medication that does not give me much relief.

Marcia D. Right now I take Vicodin and Tylenol, which are basically the only pain relievers I take. I also take Diovan for high blood pressure, Zoloft for depression, Glucovance for diabetes, Lasix for water retention, potassium, and Accolate and albuterol for asthma. I'm sure there are more I'm not remembering. I take about twelve different pills a day.

Sondra H. I monitor my medications and do not take them daily, but rather listen to my body and take them as prescribed when I feel the FM is moving into a cycle. As I explained to my doctors when treatment began, I dislike taking a lot of medication. Taking the fifteen to twenty pills a day they prescribed was very difficult, but it was something I had to do. It was scary. It's not the physical part of taking medications that bothers me, but rather the importance I place on being in tune with my body and not wanting to give it something it doesn't need.

Once again, Sondra's discussion of balancing her body's needs with following "doctor's orders" illustrates the importance of being your own advocate during treatment for a chronic condition.

COMPLEMENTARY TREATMENTS

In *Alternative Treatments for Fibromyalgia and Chronic Fatigue Syndrome*, we discussed many of the alternative, or complementary, therapies available to treat FM. A combination of both standard and alternative treatments has worked best for my symptoms. Exercise, physical therapy, and chiropractic treatment combined with medication and supplements form the building blocks of my treatment plan. I have also found that yoga, meditation, and movement therapies work and are affordable. I try new products or therapies regularly, being careful to use only those that are proven to work, either scientifically or through years of tried and true anecdotal evidence. And these days, studies are beginning to confirm what practitioners of Eastern medicine have known for centuries: that yoga, meditation, and guided imagery work to calm symptoms and help with pain relief.

This section gives a brief overview of some of the complementary therapies available to add to your treatment protocol. (See Chapter 12 for a closer look at two complementary therapies: naturopathy and energy therapy.) If you are thinking of trying chiropractic or one of the movement therapies, first read about it or find an FM friend who has had good results. Or talk with your doctor or physical therapist. Investigate any complementary therapy before you spend money on it. The same goes for supplements and exercise programs.

We all have heard the stories of the magic devices or cremes or gels that take away the pain of FM. We who endure pain and fatigue daily want relief, and we are often victims of buying the next new miracle supplement or buying into the latest fad based on dubious claims. If you're going to try alternative treatments, it is important to find one that both helps your symptoms and doesn't break your bank. Make sure it is a truly complementary therapy—that is, one that will enhance your already established plan of care.

Nearly all the women I interviewed told me they use some form of alternative or complementary therapy, so it shouldn't be hard to find other people who've tried a treatment you're considering. Ask around in your support group or in an online chat group. The website ImmuneSupport.com keeps up on the newest dietary supplements that have been tested and proven to help. Remember, start slowly, with only one therapy at a time. That way, you will know what is helping and what isn't.

An important pointer from the preceding section bears repeating: Supplements are available without a prescription, but that doesn't mean their use should be treated lightly, *especially if you're taking any prescription medications.* Some supplements are powerful drugs in their own right, and they can interfere with or complicate the effects of other drugs. Before adding any supplements to your treatment regimen, discuss the matter with either your physician or a qualified herbalist or nutritionist knowledgeable about FM.

Sondra H. I try to do the things that were taught to me at the pain clinic. I approach everything in moderation, but what works for me is yoga, walking, regular massages (this is by no means a luxury; it is often painful and a challenge, but it helps break up the knots in my muscles and is a much better alternative than shots), and, in warm weather, swimming.

Gerry L. Currently, I get acupuncture and regular massage therapy from someone who knows FM. I've also tried craniosacral release, Reiki, healing touch, hot packs, warm-water exercises taught by a physical therapist, biofeedback, cognitive therapy, supplements, pain medications, medication for delta 4 sleep, and homeopathy. Also important is honoring the body by listening to it. Rest and more rest. Music relaxation and guided relaxation. Meditation. For the first time in ten years, I am having some small success with exercise and stretching, but it is a very slow process that I must be consistent with. I have tried a grocery list of therapeutic treatments and medications that have not worked or that had terrible side effects.

I still see the same doctor. He has been studying FM for about sixteen years. He understands it. He has taught me to never apologize to pharmacists or anyone else for having to take some of the medications I need to take. I have learned that there is a place for both traditional and alternative or complementary medicine, as I like to call it.

Right now I rely on a wonderful woman who is a chiropractor, R.N., and acupuncturist. She has been treating me for several years. I must tell you, I never believed in chiropractors, but I was desperate. She has helped me more than the numerous M.D.s I have gone to over the years. Our relationship is one of complete trust and respect on both sides. She is knowledgeable and patient and cares about the whole person. She has opened doors for me.

But I was the one who made the decision to try. We have had some success. I know it would not matter to her if the person in chronic pain was a woman or man. She doesn't just listen, she hears. She has always encouraged me to look into other therapies and treatments. She will also read about and research them. We have learned a lot from each other. She has watched me shoot myself in the foot many times. She continues with dialogue; she never judges. Before her, I had never connected with a doctor in this way. And it is not only because of the remedies she uses—the heat packs, acupuncture, gentle adjustments, homeopathic supplements and herbs, etc. It is because she has helped me to learn that it is all connected—mind, body, spirit, soul. We are part of the universe. Her practice provides a place of peace and healing.

I also see a doctor who practices Chinese and traditional medicine. He is a wonderful and caring doctor. He does acupuncture and examines his patients in the Chinese fashion. He believes, as does my chiropractor, in detoxing for the yeast found in most FM patients. This proved true for me through testing. I was off the charts with yeast in my intestines. The detox caused a healing crisis, so I was quite sick with every kind of symptom you can have during a flare-up. But it turned around my IBS (irritable bowel syndrome). My chiropractor also does this; her method is a little more gentle on the body, but just as effective.

Rae H. Currently I am using Tylenol, ibuprofen, and 5-HTP (a supplement derived from the amino acid tryptophan) for sleep. The 5-HTP is wonderful—I can often sleep several hours at a time. Although I still wake up exhausted, I'm able to function better than I can without any sleep. Without the 5-HTP, I have difficulty getting to sleep, with devastating results. I've tried physical therapy (with variable results), biofeedback (helpful because I learned to relax and manage my reaction to stress), and trigger-point injections (with variable results). By far, the most helpful interventions have been "energy work" (Reiki/healing touch) and massage therapy.

Sisu G. I have tried meditation, and it helps. Nobody told me the critical rule: Don't expect to be good at this from the start. I'm up to about five minutes at a time, and I couldn't get through my mornings without that meditation break. And those wearable heating pads? Medical miracle. I love them. I use them once every week or two to get through the worst days. My work schedule begins in the early morning, when I feel best, and ends around four, just when I feel I can't go on. I do fairly well most days, but there are days when I could scream. Heat works best; I take hot baths at night two or three times a week.

Patricia S. I have closets full of supplements that I take every day. I can't begin to list them all. I've long since lost track of the number of physicians I have seen. Thirty to forty? I've also lost track of the number of treatments I've tried, including acupuncture, meditation, physical therapy, myofascial work, vegetarianism, sclerotherapy, dry needling, trigger-point injections, massage, electrotherapy, magnetic therapy, chelation, removal of mercury fillings, colonics, countless supplements, hormone therapy, and many others I can't remember. Many I didn't really believe in based on my Western medical training, but I am desperate to keep an open mind. I do my research and decide whether or not it's just too nuts to try. I feel if it doesn't hurt me, what have I got to lose? Sometimes when I try something now I am afraid, second guessing, wondering how it will help me. Am I being something akin to ethnocentric about my knowledge? We don't know everything yet, that's for sure. Anyway, some of the therapies do help me a bit, but nothing really gets its teeth into the syndrome. It still remains and makes my life miserable.

Donna F. Many treatments are available to manage pain. I didn't want to get into a treatment I knew I couldn't continue or benefit from. I turned away from massage therapy primarily because of inconvenience and cost. I do moderate stretching. On good days, my exercise is walking. I cannot do any exercise that is too strenuous because of the payoff, which includes heart problems, lots of Achilles pain, extreme exhaustion, and an enormous toll of stress on my muscles. I just started seeing a chiropractor, and that helps a great deal. Watching what I eat and drink is a battle, but it helps lessen heart problems and achiness, I am told. I sincerely believe that if I didn't take anything to control my heart problems associated with the condition, I would not be here for much longer. At one point I thought my days were numbered. The heart problems had really altered my involvement with my family because of their intensity and unpredictability. I would have to close myself alone in my room away from any noise or activity just to relieve the chest pain, difficulty breathing, and fiercely pounding heart.

Jean T. I saw an advertisement for the Alpha Stim 100 on the Internet. It is a microcurrent and cranial electrotherapy stimulator. The doctor gave me a prescription to get one. I use it for one hour each morning, and afterward all of the deep bone pain is gone. It stays gone for the entire day unless a big storm is coming in. In that case I usually use it again for fifteen minutes or so, and it works. I really think the combination of the Alpha Stim and the Prozac is keeping me feeling so much better. I sure wouldn't part with them.

Donnie M. One of the best things I use for pain is a TENS unit (see page 94). Without it my life would be much worse. It has allowed me to be more active and get out of bed and off the heating pad. I also use magnet therapy for energy. At first I thought it was stupid, but I was wrong. It does not help my pain, only my energy level. Of course, I do not have the energy I had when I was not sick, but at least I can function a little more with the use of the magnets. I don't even begin to understand how it works. I just know it has helped me a little. I have to do anything I can to survive FM.

Val T. I get water therapy from a hot tub I purchased a few months ago, and the results are amazing. I use it at least every other day. I have a caudal (an epidural injection to block back pain) roughly once every four months for the extreme back pain, and that gives me a lot of relief. I also get trigger-point injections as needed.

I would also suggest therapeutic touch. It is a great way to relax and get much-needed sleep and pain relief. I was taught the technique in nursing school, and I have heard many great stories of its benefits on TV as well as seeing it with my own eyes. My instructor at the time told us students about a patient in the hospital dying from cancer. No amount of pain medication ever allowed her any relief to sleep. My instructor and her colleagues spent several hours doing therapeutic touch on this woman, and her pain totally subsided. She slept for almost twenty-four hours, the first time in days without pain. The hospital pharmacy could not believe how well she responded without the use of narcotics.

Therapeutic touch involves directing electrical energy by either touching the person or by standing less than an arm's length from them and sweeping outwards over different areas of their bodies. An analogy is a tree whose branches cannot receive the needed nutrients and water. Practitioners of therapeutic touch believe that the "branches," or energy pathways, throughout the body are plugged; moving the electrical energy through them opens them up to receive better circulation, thus relieving pain and relaxing the body.

Lindamarie M. I found that the Feldenkrais Method helped a lot. My perception became clearer, and I had fewer headaches and an increase in mobility. Other therapies have helped me in many different ways, including putting me in remission for about a year from 1999 to 2000—lymphatic drainage, Reiki, massage therapy, yoga, breathing work, and creative dance therapy/movement. Since Medicare doesn't cover these treatments, I could not afford to maintain them. I never considered myself to be "giving up" on this list of therapies; it's just that money is a huge factor in treatment.

Emma L. Therapeutic swimming and gentle shiatsu-type massage help a lot. Chiropractic helped with the stiffness in the neck and shoulders and did a lot to relieve carpal tunnel pain. Nothing consistently helps with fatigue. Pet animals have helped with loneliness.

Victoria M. I have tried many herbal treatments, injections into trigger points, chiropractic treatments, and taking large doses of individual vitamins, which I have given up. I have eliminated certain food types, mainly gluten, and reduced consumption of possible irritants such as coffee and sugar. Two weeks ago I began using the supplement SAM-e and will continue with it. I also drink plenty of filtered water and get regular rest. I am mindful that I need to monitor my activity level, and to make sure I look after myself, physically and emotionally.

Cheryl R. I get chiropractic deep-heat therapy and interferential treatments (which involve electrical stimulation of nerves and surrounding tissues) every other week, and I have for four years. I have tried so many drugs that didn't work, I couldn't list them all. But now I'm on a combination of prescriptions that seems to be working. I tried acupuncture and it made my pain worse. I have also tried overhead traction and pain clinics (a real joke). One more thing that does not work is a doctor who doesn't support you. I've found that the way to get by is to take my meds and pray, and to try to live one day at a time.

▲▲▲

Whatever treatment options you and your health-care team decide you should try, remember that taking good care of yourself is the most important part of your life now. Don't give up on finding ways to lessen the pain of FM. The women I have met who are now in remission have found the right combination of medication, supplements, rest, exercise, and some type of positive mind control, whether it be meditation, self-hypnosis, energy work, or prayer.

Another important characteristic these women have in common is that they view FM as a *part* of their life, not its focus. For most people with chronic illness, arriving at such an attitude doesn't happen overnight. First on the emotional agenda is coming to terms with what we've lost and dealing with the accompanying feelings of anger and depression—that is, grieving. This is the topic of the next chapter.

Our Mental and Emotional Health

More and more health professionals are getting it that fibromyalgia is not "all in your head." The myth of the "FM personality" has been proven unfounded. Conferences are held every year or so where we can listen to doctors and researchers speak about the newest fibromyalgia theories and treatments. Support groups exist in hospitals and chat rooms. All of these advances in support for FM patients can help us deal with the depression, anger, grief, and loss that inevitably accompany any chronic-pain condition.

When I was diagnosed with FM in 1993, the first book I read was one about chronic fatigue syndrome (with which I was also diagnosed), *Running on Empty* (recently revised and retitled *Chronic Fatigue Syndrome, Fibromyalgia, and Other Invisible Illnesses*), by Katrina Berne, Ph.D. I read it as fast as I could, soaking in the information. Armed with that book, my two diagnoses, and my Arthritis Foundation pamphlets, I went out and found a support group. It was there, among women like myself, that I explored the strong emotions that arose because my life had been so completely changed.

All of the women interviewed for this book expressed similar emotions. And why not? If you have FM, chances are you've been faced with feeling like you've had the flu for months or years, with aching all over, with experiencing myriad confusing symptoms, yet also with having a very difficult time getting a diagnosis, and then with having to explain your condition to family and friends, who may or may not understand. Depression, anger, and feelings of loss are very normal under circumstances such as these. This chapter relates women's experiences with these emotions and discusses ways of dealing with them.

DEPRESSION

As anyone who suffers from depression can tell you, the condition is very difficult to explain to someone who has never known it. To me it's like being underwater where it's dark and I am alone, while everyone else is on the shore playing, reading, sitting in the sun, enjoying life. Nothing seems very important anymore, and sleep is an escape that beckons me during all my waking hours. Those are the bad days.

Back in the mid-1980s, I remember filling out the paperwork for a weekend seminar about changing your life. This particular seminar was presented in nearly every big city; it came and went under different names for over thirty years. One of the questions I answered (before I paid my several hundred dollars to be deprived of food, rest, and a bathroom break) was, "Are you winning at therapy?" It was a question I couldn't answer then, but I can do so now.

For the last eighteen years, I have seen a therapist, a new one every few years. If I'd saved up all the money I have spent talking about my life, I could buy a really loaded SUV, but therapy for me has been priceless. It always made perfect sense to me to take good care of my mental health as well as my physical health. When my everyday depression turned into clinical depression and then rapidly escalated into suicidal thoughts and a plan, I knew I had to get additional help. The simple act of making a call to my doctor brought me back. Extra visits to my therapists were required to get me through that rough patch. It wasn't easy.

Serious depression is a challenge that must be worked on every day. A long time ago, before I had FM, one of my therapists asked me what I did when I couldn't move because of depression. I answered, "I just try to do *one* thing." It's advice I still follow. That one thing might be getting up and watering my plants. Or eating something, since I tend not to eat when I am depressed. Or taking a shower. The decision to get up and get moving seems to help lift the depression enough to motivate me to do one more thing.

I worked on a crisis hotline for thirteen months during the second year after my diagnosis with FM. I am so glad I volunteered my time. I learned to recognize the sounds of a depressed person and an imminently suicidal one. I learned about the treatment and services available for a person who is fighting depression and loss. If you have suffered from depression, then you probably have a few tricks in your bag for dealing with it. Calling a friend works for some women; exercising helps others. But if you're struggling with depression, do something. Take action. Depression can be the fight of your life. We all know stories about people who couldn't take the pain and depression anymore and ended their lives. Before you get to that place, *call someone.* Don't try to handle such feelings alone. Nearly every community has a crisis hotline; you can find the number in your local phone book.

Depression and FM

I've spoken with many women who suffer from depression along with fibromyalgia. Some of the symptoms of the two conditions, such as fatigue and sleep difficulties, are similar. Several sources estimate that approximately 25 percent of FM patients have clinical depression. It's not such a big step to imagine this of a person who has been leading a normal life, has a job and family and friends they love, and then—WHAM!—they're in a car accident, and the resulting FM changes everything. Who wouldn't be depressed?

Fortunately, the stigma of depression has been broken because of recognition of its seriousness by medical professionals, the willingness of public personalities to speak about the condition, and the success of new drugs like Prozac and Effexor. Antidepressants are often prescribed for FM. These drugs can help with sleep, pain, *and* depression. Be up-front with your doctor; tell him or her about your symptoms of depression. In addition to pharmaceuticals, many natural remedies exist for treating depression, and don't forget that regular exercise can help. You can't separate the mind from the body, so why treat only one?

To deal with the almost inevitable feelings of loss and depression that accompany a diagnosis of FM or any other serious chronic illness, you must have a support system in place. It could be a friend or your partner, a support group or a therapist. Read about some of our correspondents' support networks in Chapters 3 and 8. Whatever you choose, find someone you trust and can talk to about the pain and fatigue of FM, and about your feelings around having a chronic illness. If the idea of therapy makes you feel uncomfortable, start with an FM support group. But nothing substitutes for good one-on-one therapy; think of it as the mental-health part of your treatment plan.

On an average day, I can distinguish between FM symptoms and depression, and I usually can control the depression quite well. But like everyone else with chronic pain, I have to be determined to fight it. I recognize—and I'll bet you do too—the difference between the depression I experienced before FM and the type I experience now. Having a chronic-pain condition—being in pain every day, twenty-four hours a day—takes every ounce of strength you have. Consequently, with FM, depression now may come on a bit more readily and may last a bit longer.

But I'll repeat: If your depression gets out of hand, you *must* get help right away. Don't downplay your symptoms, and don't try to "wait it out," especially if you are thinking of suicide. If you exhibit any of the following signs, there's a good chance your depression has advanced from the normal depression that accompanies a life-changing loss, such as diagnosis with FM, and has turned into clinical depression. *If this list or part of this list describes you, help is out there. Get some.*

Signs of Clinical Depression

◀ Noticeable change in eating habits. Some women eat more when they are depressed. Or the opposite may apply: Their appetite just isn't there; food might seem tasteless and like too much of a bother to prepare.

◀ Changes in sleep patterns. Some women sleep more and don't want to get up in the morning. Or they can't fall asleep because they're thinking about their problems.

◀ Withdrawing from family, friends, and work. It may seem like your circle of friends doesn't understand what is happening to you and your family. You may feel as though the best thing to do is to be alone.

◀ Difficulty concentrating. Feelings of sadness and loss seem to take over your thoughts.

◀ Thoughts of suicide, and maybe a plan for how to carry it out.

Marcia D. I found out from the psychiatrist that I have a form of clinical depression called dysthymia. It is very treatable as long as I stay on my medication. I have tried, at times, to go off the medication, but the longest I've been off it is six weeks; then I had to go back on it. They told me it is a lifelong condition. I will probably be on medication the rest of my life.

When I am depressed, I have a tendency to not leave the house. I don't talk to people. I don't want to be around people. If I do something like grocery shopping, I usually do it early in the morning or late at night. I don't like to put myself in a position that would really stress me out, so I control what I do and where I go. This doesn't make my husband happy, because he is a very people-oriented person, but I need to do it to take care of myself.

Denise P. I guess what I feel most of the time is depression. It's not so bad, however, that I let it get me down. I don't have anyone living close by who is really there for me when I need someone. I have a close friend at work, but we don't see a lot of each other outside of work. My daughter is only twenty, with a baby, and doesn't understand what I go through. I have a boyfriend, but he has his own health problems and doesn't understand what I go through and isn't interested in finding out.

Donna P. When I was first diagnosed with FM, my world crumbled. No more working, and believe me I tried to keep working, but it was just too much. I became depressed and lost interest in everything. Basically I wanted to die. I ended up in the mental ward. FM and several other horrific things were the cause.

Alison H. Sadness and depression are things I fight almost daily. It's hard to look around at people doing the things I want to do and have to just sit back and watch. It's hard to know that people see me as different and sometimes as lazy. It's hard to have to evaluate every action before I can do it. I hate it that people have to rearrange plans for me. I hate it that I have had to reevaluate my life's goals, because it's uncertain whether I will be able to do all of the things I wanted to do. I am angered that I may be unable to go through normal childbirth because I don't know if I can handle the pain. There are times when I feel so alone and so lost. It's this deep, empty feeling that is hard to ignore.

However, there are also times when I am grateful for all I've gone through. Because of my experiences, I will be able to be there for others who are going through the same thing. I can help someone else to feel less alone than I did at first.

LOW SELF-ESTEEM

Self-esteem can suffer when your life is dramatically changed by a chronic-pain condition. When you are unable to keep up with family and friends, and going to the doctor happens more often than going out and having fun, your self-esteem can take a beating.

Lalenya R. Pre-FM, I was active, slim, happy. I sometimes don't understand why I can't "beat" this thing. I've lived with adversity before, and I've always made the best of it. But with this condition, I've gained weight and feel like an old woman.

Cydney B. My self-esteem has taken a real battering. My self-satisfaction and my self-actualization have suffered. I am not who I thought I was going to be. I am not who I want my children (both women) to see as their mom.

Now is the time to remind yourself that you are still the same person you always were, even though some medications may cause weight gain or loss, or losing ground in your exercise program may show up on your body. In the beginning, a positive body image can be hard to hold onto when you are in pain, but you must try your hardest to keep your spirits up. Don't fall into negative self-talk. It might sound like a small voice in your head that says, "I'm not as firm and trim as I once was. I can't do the fun things I used to. Life is passing me by." Stop that voice! Doing so takes practice; really pay attention to the thoughts that slip fleetingly through your mind. Whenever you notice a piece of negative self-talk, replace it with a positive truth about your life, called an *affirmation*. Here are some examples: "My pain is a little less intense today than it was yesterday." Or, "The sun filtering through the trees in my backyard is so beautiful." Or, "My life is incredibly blessed with the love of family and friends." Find the positive in your daily life. It's there in the faces of your loved ones, the silky fur of your pets, and your spiritual faith. If affirmations seem too much like sugarcoating your problems, it works for some people to simply breathe deeply several times, while focusing their thoughts on a quality they want more of in their life, such as peace, joy, or beauty. Sometimes just breathing deeply while repeating a word such as *peace, joy,* or *beauty* over and over silently, like a mantra, can shift your frame of mind in a matter of seconds.

However you do it, recognize that today's pain and exhaustion may be different tomorrow. I tell myself that the pain and fatigue always pass, and I find ways of getting my mind off of them. One of the things I do to keep my spirits up is to avoid focusing on the pain. I try not to talk about my illness unless asked directly about

it. Or embrace a goal unrelated to your illness. Start with something easy, like getting a donation together for a local thrift store—
anything to take your mind away from the pain.

Here are some more ideas:

Things to Do When Your Self-Esteem Is Low

◀ Watch a funny video or sitcom on TV.

◀ Play with children. If you don't have kids, borrow the
neighbor's. There are four children in my neighborhood
whom I always enjoy watching. They are still young
enough to think I'm cool.

◀ Do something kind for someone. This always helps me.
Even if it's just cutting some flowers for your neighbor, it
gets your focus off the pain for a minute.

◀ Find the mirror and look at the best part of your body.
Remind yourself you are still the same woman you were
before FM. Shamelessly ask your husband or partner to list
the beautiful parts about you. This may surprise you! The
list probably won't all be about your body.

◀ Pray, meditate, or write in your journal.

If you don't know where to start with any one of these practices, begin by being thankful for what is positive in your life.
Doing so will become easier after a while. When my partner did
this, I had a peek at her list. It said, "I am thankful for my soft covers and quilt. I am thankful for my dogs and kitties, and I am
happy that Mari feels better today." Wow! Those words trans-
formed me. Now I try to think of my own gratitudes every night. A
famous talk-show host swears that if you write down five things
each night that you are grateful for from your day—things specific
to that day, like "I love the new haircut I got today," rather than
generic things, like being thankful for your home, family, and food
on the table—your life will soon change for the better.

STRESS

The phones are ringing. It's 10:00 A.M. on a busy workday. I am the only employee in the store; the other florist is late. There are orders to finish for delivery and boxes of flowers to clean before the arrangements can be made. The doorbell chimes, and a customer comes in to complain that her gift of roses died the day after she ordered them. I look in the file and the original order is missing...

The above is a good example of a stressful situation from my old life. Back then, before fibromyalgia, I might have gotten a bit nervous and maybe sweated a little. But within the next few hours I would have had the energy to settle the situation with the customer and then gone on to each task and completed them one by one.

Now stress looks a lot different and can send me into a tailspin. It can be triggered by something like having a doctor's appointment, running late, and then realizing that my car is out of gas. Chronic pain takes a lot of energy to fight. Simple tasks that once were manageable seem impossible if you are exhausted and in pain. Nowadays, my life is pared down to avoid stress. But getting rid of stress entirely? Not possible. Unforeseen events will always pop up. It's a fact of life. The key is keeping those stressful situations from overwhelming you. Here are some ideas for doing so:

Tips for Reducing Stress

◀ Plan your day carefully to avoid overdoing it (see Chapter 7 for more on this topic).

◀ Ask for help when you need it.

◀ Use exercise, meditation, and guided imagery for stress reduction.

◀ Do less each day than you think you are capable of. Conserve your energy.

◀ Remember to include pleasurable activities in your day.

Katie G. A life stressor for me would be trying to do too much in a day, or overscheduling. Consequently, I have had to break ties with some people because they were negative, unsupportive, or even jealous. Another stressor would be failing to get my exercise in, because it does help! I try to structure each day and make it as productive as possible. I am goal-oriented, and I go at my own pace. Writing a list and crossing off each item completed gives me a sense of accomplishment.

I no longer work, and it's stressful to be asked if I'm working or when I will go back to work, etc. If asked, I take a deep breath and say I'm working on my health or on getting into remission. I also do some volunteer work, which is immensely gratifying.

Val T. Stress is a part of all our lives, and a lot of it cannot be controlled, such as the stress from family members, work, keeping up a house, and fighting the daily struggles with fatigue and pain. To eliminate stress entirely, you'd need to divorce yourself from everyone and everything, which is impossible! I have found that a lot of FM patients suffer with stress and always want to take on the whole world. They feel responsible for many things that are not in their control. They are the "fixers" of the world.

My life stressors include holding down my jobs and keeping my life organized, as well as housework—cooking, cleaning, laundry, and bills. My family relationships are another stressor, as is getting enough sleep. Of course, the biggest stressor is the pain and the effort involved in trying to remain pain-free.

Since my illness began, I have tried to control my stress levels, because I experienced a definite increase in pain each time I felt myself getting stressed. In the mornings I would cry and be angry because I couldn't move right away and the pain was so severe. But getting upset only made things worse. After a while I caught on to what I was doing, so instead I would simply lie there and relax, thinking of other things or turning on my favorite radio station. Other things I tried for relaxation included jumping into a warm whirlpool bath with my favorite scents, reading, enjoying an infrared sauna, and massage. I purchased several meditation tapes to fall asleep by. (I bought a portable cassette player and soft earplugs that wouldn't bother me while I slept.) The tapes knocked me out almost immediately. Reflexology and therapeutic touch also helped.

I adjusted my work hours, but work continues to be a huge stress factor. On my days off I often stress out from fear that I will hurt really badly the next day while I'm working. I've learned to receive help with the cleaning and cooking, but I often feel guilty when I can't cook a meal for my family after work or on bad days. I do my best to keep plans I have made with family members. The guilt of not doing things seems to be worse than just carrying through with the plans. I have strong feelings that I will not let my family suffer just because I suffer. I realize this creates stress, but my love for them is most important and my driving force.

I cue myself when I first notice that my stress level is high, and I try to calm down before I pay for it. This is the biggest feat I have to accomplish.

Marcia D. I am probably one of a million women who grew up, got married, had kids, took care of a house, took care of a husband, and held down a job. I was basically doing three or four jobs in one lifetime. I think somewhere along the line, if you don't handle stress well, then pretty soon something goes "bang" and the body starts fighting against itself. I think the body can only take so much emotional and physical stress, and then it has to give.

Carol J. Life stressors are an ongoing battle. Becoming single, being out of a job, caring for a child alone, having to apply for disability, and adjusting to life with little income have been the biggest problems I've faced. I've dealt with them, and now my stress level has dropped from over nine hundred to around one hundred on the stress chart, so I have progressed.

Penny G. Perfectionism is my stressor. I keep telling myself that I am fine and do not have to be perfect and please everyone. I have issues with family members. I choose not to spend time with family members unless I feel very strong emotionally. My weight is also a stressor. I weigh about 170 pounds, whereas I should be at 120–130 pounds. I am dealing with that slowly, by eating nutritiously and forgiving myself for being fat. I also take on way too much, but I am learning to say no. I am taking on only those activities that I truly love, and I am letting others do the rest.

Mary H.-B. I have been able to identify my stressors, and I work daily in meditation on the issues that cause me stress. I work on saying no to negativity in my life.

Cydney B. Work stressed me. But I think I liked it. It had good and bad implications. I was so busy, working sixty- to seventy-hour weeks. My husband and I used to laugh and say we needed to hire a mother to take care of us because we no longer had time to take care of ourselves.

The first year I stopped working, it was just hell. I had a new idea every day for some great job I could do at home. Drove my husband nuts. After a few years that died down. I actually did do some part-time work in an area I'd always wanted to work in—journalism. And now, I don't know how I ever did all that working, even healthy! I deal with the loss of self-esteem that I had when I worked by discouraging myself from getting caught up in that form of self-definition. I am more "me" than I may have been as an "overachiever."

But now being sick stresses me. Not that I am worried about impending death or complete disability, but rather that I can't meet my own or others' expectations or needs anymore. I want to be able to exercise, travel, go places when I want, make plans and be able to keep them, support my children emotionally and physically if they need me, and be a wife to my husband and not depend on him to do the "woman" things around the house. I am still dealing with those stressors and haven't found nirvana yet. Have you? If so, please tell me how.

▲▲▲

ANGER AND RESENTMENT

My therapist tells me that fear is at the bottom of every situation in which I feel angry. So far, she's been right. I started out being afraid at the pain clinic where the young doctor hurt me during an examination, but I went away *mad*! Mad that he didn't "hear" me when I told him he was pressing way too hard on the tender points. Mad that several of the doctors treated me with disrespect and disbelief. And mad that I received no help at all. I wrote about this incident in *Alternative Treatments for Fibromyalgia and Chronic Fatigue Syndrome*. It was the worst doctor experience I've ever had. But it goes right to the center of what made me the angriest about having fibromyalgia: I look fine on the outside; FM is an invisible illness. Right after diagnosis, this was my first big hurdle.

In the beginning, it meant everything when family and friends and even folks I had just met understood—really got it—what FM was, from the pain to the cognitive dysfunction. I was mad that I couldn't work and earn money. I was furious that I had to stay home during the day while my friends' lives went on as usual. But mainly it was the illness itself. No one in my group of friends or family had heard about it, and it seemed to me that people just didn't believe me when I said I had FM.

Then there was the anger directed at myself for all the things I could no longer do. Every FM patient knows that if you want or need desperately to get something done, you can do it. It's a matter of how much it will cost you the next day in terms of pain and exhaustion. I still get mad when I think that friends or family members only see me out and about when I am the best I can be for an event. They don't know what it costs me later on. Most of the time I don't let the "costs" bother me, because I will not let FM run my life. I am participating no matter what! I don't go around talking about my illness in a way that lets everyone know the details. But sometimes when folks say, "You look great! I am glad to see how much better you are! When are you returning to work?"—aaagh!

We have all heard the advice to release anger by pounding on pillows with a stick or throwing rocks into the ocean. My friend's favorite trick is to buy old used dishes at a garage sale and throw them against a wall. This method is easy to clean up and doesn't hurt anything. Or she breaks cheap Christmas-tree balls against a cement floor. Again, doing this is cheap and doesn't destroy anything of value. And the shattering of something breakable is so effective.

I am a cleaner. When I feel angry, I clean my house. Still, too many times I have yelled and hurt someone I love. When that happens I try to remind myself that getting the anger and resentment out is about feeling better, not about hurting someone else. Equally as often, I must remind myself to treat *myself* gently. It's easy to be harder on ourselves than on anyone else.

It's helpful to remember the advice of health experts who point out that anger and resentment don't do us much good in the long run. If you hold onto your feelings of anger and resentment, you won't move forward. In the short run, anger may motivate you to make some good changes, and when those changes are accomplished, it's time to let go of the anger.

If you find that you are angry and resentful most of the time, try to:

◀ find out what you are most angry about,

◀ decide if there is anything you can do about it,

◀ make any changes you think might be beneficial—don't stew in those strong emotions.

Remember, anger and resentment can control you, and being angry won't help your FM. Resenting the fact that you have the illness won't cure it. Let those two difficult emotions go. You will feel better for it!

Patricia S. I am very angry. I've lost so much of my life—the work, the play, the intimacy. It is terribly frustrating. And then to not be taken seriously by most people is the frosting on the cake. I want to scream and throw things at people. It doesn't make sense that this illness should be so mysterious and that patients should have to lobby to get attention paid to it. I am very angry at my medical colleagues.

In addition, I do get scared when I have a strong exacerbation, with the constant burning, the inability to sit comfortably, have sex, ride a bicycle. It gives me great grief. It's pain that drives one nuts. I fear that this state will become my baseline and I'll have to learn to live like this. When I get a gynecological infection, I am terrified that the pain will never go away, and I become anxious and depressed. Even just thinking about the pain of my original infection makes me anxious and I start to cry. Some might call this post-traumatic stress disorder. It does feel that profound.

My life stressors are no different from anyone else's. I have to learn to "not sweat the small stuff." When we get angry, we usually get tense. That tension only makes the muscles hurt more. I have to learn to better handle the situations that get me angry and seek to change them instead of just being angry.

Donnie M. I am mad as hell. I feel very alone and as though no one cares, and I do so wish they did care. I want to say I am not scared, but maybe I am, as I never know what new problem brought on by FM will hit me next. I am very short on patience with others; it makes me angry to see them doing and enjoying all the things I can never do again. FM has taken my life away from me. It is in control, not me.

Rachel B. I was so angry because I didn't envision myself living like this. I'm tired of fighting a battle against an invisible disease that, in the end, I feel I'm losing. I'm scared for my job and my future capabilities. I know someone else who has FM, but our symptoms don't really match. That adds to my feelings of aloneness. I resent that I have to rely upon others to help me, since I feel I'm losing my independence. I know that I easily put up my protective wall, so that when people ask me how I'm feeling, I quickly resort to the "I'm okay, I'm fine" attitude. I do not want FM to interfere with my life and with what I want to accomplish.

Rae H. I am furious. I believe there is a strong link between historical trauma and FM. I've done a lot of work around my emotional healing and believe I have done a great job with it. To have my physical body still "under attack" seems terribly unfair. I find FM to be very isolating because of the lack of energy to tend to high-maintenance friendships. Between the time and energy pressures of work, the book I'm writing, husband, and home, there just isn't much left to allow me to participate more fully in friendships and be active in my church. We live in the country and I can't see to drive at night, so I've been disappointed (and disappointing) in my inability to attend even the most basic of evening activities. I struggle to separate depression from fibro fog, and I struggle with recognizing that a lack of wanting to get out of bed means I am truly exhausted rather than depressed.

Ginger C. I feel angry at times, angry that I have to put up with this illness. I also feel frustrated and alone. Family and friends try to understand and help, but sometimes I feel they just can't understand what it is like to endure constant pain and fatigue. My husband wants me to talk to him about it, but I find that very hard to do. I don't want to seem as if I am always complaining about FM. Some days, I just feel depressed and want to cry, and I don't know why.

Penny G. I am very angry about getting this stupid illness. I feel that I had enough challenges growing up and that I deserve better. I hate being in pain and feeling angry about it. I am scared of getting worse and depending more on others. I feel alone because I look pretty healthy, so everyone assumes I am fine; thus, I don't feel I belong anywhere—not with the healthy people and not with those who are disabled and unable to work. I resent all the time I lose when I am in pain. On the other hand, I feel some positive gratitude when people do understand and help me in a way that does not feel demeaning.

Gina H. I'm mad, I'm scared, and I feel alone. I just don't know what to expect. What I resent the most is when doctors treat us like a basket of rolls being passed around at dinner. Because they don't believe in FM, they send us from one doctor to another and give us medicine for depression because they cannot heal us. Sometimes I feel I just can't take it any more, so thoughts of suicide have come up. But I just remember the mustard seed in the *Bible* and continue to carry one. Every day I write in my journal about my day, and if I feel all right, I talk to my support group.

Mary H.-B. I'm not mad anymore, nor am I scared. I don't feel alone, either. I resent that no one really wants to listen when you try to explain what is going on in your body on a daily basis. They are too wrapped up in themselves to listen. They just look at me and see that I look fine and form the opinion that I'm lying.

Denise P. I am mad about having FM. I'm only fifty-three, and it's as if my body is aging ten times as fast as it should. My twin sister doesn't have any of the health problems that I have, and I guess that makes me angry—not with her but with life. Why me? I'm really scared about what my health will be like five to ten years from now. I am really alone. I'm tired of hurting all the time and would like someone to share all of it with. I don't know if my boyfriend and I will ever live together. I would like to live with him and be able to share with him. Some days, the pain is so bad I can hardly get out of bed. On those days I can't even walk.

Cydney B. I resent that the entire course of my life has been altered from what I had envisioned all my adult life. It makes me really mad.

I also know I am unbelievably blessed to have had the structures in place to make this blow have a minimal impact on me, financially and emotionally. To have become more dependent on someone would have been much more devastating. To have had a truly considerable downturn in my lifestyle would have been devastating and to have that affect my children would have been awful as well. My life has been one blessed save after another, and so far it hasn't stopped. I am somewhat awed by this, and grateful.

▲▲▲

GRIEF AND LOSS

Every once in a while a huge wave of loss crashes over me—usually when I smell lilacs or roses or when it's Christmastime. When folks start putting little white lights on their houses and colorful wreaths on their doors, I get squeezed around my heart and I miss my old job. It was a career really, the only job I ever stayed at for more than a few months. I stayed thirteen years. But I'm still a florist at heart.

Those of you who have lost your jobs to FM know what I mean. Suddenly there is no reason to get out of bed at five A.M. If you were a morning person, like I was, you miss the cool air and the sunrise and the aloneness of being up early. I miss having a place to go every day and the camaraderie of my work family. The women and men I worked with knew me better than my own family, and I knew their private lives inside out. One night, when I still had a pile of orders to complete for Mother's Day, I asked the two men I was working with to help keep me alert and focused by telling me a story about themselves, one I didn't know already. We shared with each other the sort of late-night stories one can bribe a coworker with once the "high" of exhaustion and holiday excitement have passed!

Adjusting to a new life, one filled with doctor's appointments, physical therapy, taking care of yourself, and time spent alone, is a difficult job. But it's just that: It's your job. You're working on your remission.

Recently, an FM friend talked to me about feeling grief all over again, even though she was diagnosed with FM years before. I reminded her, as I remind myself, that the stages of grief seem to cycle around every so often. Grief has come to me again while writing this book. I had to remind myself that I have chronic pain and I can't do everything I want to do all at once. Yet I also had to remind myself that if I didn't have FM, I wouldn't be writing this book. Some days, the only thing that gets me by is thinking of the women I have met who handle their illness with courage and grace. The loss I feel is simply about the fact that I can't write sitting down or on a computer. I am unable to work for more than an hour at a time. But I can do the things I love if I parcel out my time, conserve energy, and take care of myself. Yes, grief and loss are part of the cycle of chronic illness. When you understand that, somehow it seems easier to pass through each stage.

Women have told me of losing their careers, homes, and even partners due to FM. It's a fact that relationships can suffer when one partner becomes ill and the other partner has to step up and fill in.

Sisu G. I went through a phase of being extremely lonely and unhappy. A lot of people get put on antidepressants at that point, which is a real mistake because it doesn't address the underlying issues of grief and loss. If you don't deal with those, you'll be facing them for a very long time.

Cydney B. If you were to ask me the question "What do you miss most?" I'd answer by saying I miss my mind the most. I had a high IQ growing up. I defined myself mostly by my intellect, rather than my looks. I never thought I was particularly good-looking, although I did okay in the whole "attracting men" thing. I found it difficult to make women friends because of my intellect and my career success. And then one day in 1992, I got stupid. I mean really stupid. And after a while my boss kept telling me, "There's something wrong with your head! Ask the doctor what's going on. There's something wrong with your head!"—meaning with my intellectual level. Nothing could have been more devastating.

Gina H. The positive side is that I believe God has a plan for us. I have been wanting to write a book for years, and now look at me. Even though I can only type using one finger of one hand, I believe God has a plan for me. My mother told me that God is not going to heal everybody, so I am looking at this illness from that perspective. Still, I feel angry and sad, because I had a plan, too.

Emma L. The life stressor that has impacted me most has been giving up activities I loved, such as hiking the hills or the bay, dancing until 2:00 A.M., making friends, going places. There is no way to deal with these losses other than letting go.

Rachel B. Going from competing in triathlons, mountaineering, mountain biking, sea lifeguarding, and waterskiing to a much different type of physical exertion, such as yoga or archery, is hard to accept, especially when you are used to pushing your body to the limit. With FM, just getting through a day of work can be a challenge at times.

Victoria M. I resent the social, emotional, vocational, financial, and academic costs of this illness, including the lost dreams for my children and myself and all we had planned as a family.

Katie G. I regret that I may never live up to all the potential I had in the areas of career, activities, lifestyle, and travel. I feel severed from these things, and I grieve the lost potential.

ABUSE AND TRAUMA

As I've mentioned, over the years I've spoken to more than a hundred people who have fibromyalgia. Most of them can pinpoint an event or events that triggered the onset of their illness. Whether they have post-traumatic FM resulting from a car accident, a fall, or some other type of trauma or primary FM that comes on over time, it seems that the link between trauma and FM is accepted.

Dr. Kim Dupree-Jones, of Oregon Health & Science University, offers this theory as to why such a great proportion of FM sufferers have a history of abuse or trauma in their lives:

> FM patients may have a maladaptation of the stress response as theorized by Hans Selye, i.e., the fight-or-flight response. There are some people who have a genetic predisposition to getting fibromyalgia and who have had stressful things happen in their life—an accident, a prolonged illness, prolonged abuse by a trusted person, familial alcoholism, or living in some sort of very stressful environment. Basically, their stress-response system goes into overdrive and then is worn out. Once they're in overdrive, we think a series of proteins triggers the genetic predisposition and they will develop the syndrome.
>
> You need to have a genetic predisposition to get this illness, just like you need to have a genetic predisposition to get diabetes; there are a lot of people who weigh three hundred pounds, for example, and who eat a terrible diet but who never get diabetes. There are people who smoke cigarettes every day of their life who don't get cancer. Likewise, there are people who survive physical and psychological stresses and don't develop fibromyalgia.

In this chapter women share openly about trauma and abuse they've experienced. Sexual abuse is a topic that comes up many times. This woman writes, on condition of anonymity, about what happened to her as a little girl:

I was abused when I was around seven years old. Something ugly, inappropriate, and unpleasant was done to me by someone I loved and looked up to. This person betrayed me. He used guilt: "If you really love me...." There was a difference between us of about six years in age. The incident caused my father, normally a loving, gentle man whom I loved, to exhibit violent behavior, which I witnessed. Because I'd told what had happened, I believed the violence took place because of me. I also believed the whole thing was my fault. My mother and I sat in the dark in the next room while my father's physical punishment of the perpetrator took place. We were crying. Only I wasn't sure if she was crying for me or for the person being punished. I was never comforted or told that I did nothing wrong, that it was not my fault.

I was also terrorized in other ways, mentally and emotionally. I grew up afraid of almost everything. I was shy, small, and frail, the neat, perfect little girl trying every way I knew how to please my mother and to figure out why she always seemed to be angry at me. I used to beat my dolls. I guess they couldn't fight back.

The second time I was abused happened when I was around twenty. It was the summer before my wedding. Though shocked and frightened, I said no to what the perpetrator wanted me to do with him. It made me sick. I got out of the house. After both incidents, my memory was a blank during the days and weeks that followed. Life went on as normal. But I wonder how we just moved on.

One of the saddest feelings I have is that I did not grow up feeling safe, secure, and protected. To this day I am still afraid of the dark. And, although I treasure my quiet time, sometimes I am afraid to be alone. I hate the night, and I sleep as much as I want to. Sleep does not come easily for those of us with fibromyalgia.

Whether someone underwent a rape, child molestation, inappropriate behavior, or any other kind of physical, mental, verbal, or emotional abuse and threat, they are left with deep, sometimes festering wounds. For some, our bodies—our muscles and cells—hold these memories no matter how many years have passed, and we numb them out and push them down inside until they make us very sick.

No matter the type of abuse or trauma you may have suffered as a child or as an adult, there is no doubt it took its toll on your body and emotions. It's never too late to let these memories out in a safe and secure location with a trusted counselor or friend.

Norah T. Children who are abused can't show it, can't let anybody know. They've been told "don't tell." Because of this basic denial of themselves and their experiences, as children or adults some of them have an incredibly hard time identifying any physical illness, and the medical community reinforces that phenomenon. I am working with a Vietnam vet who suffered abuse early in his childhood, and it has taken him until five years ago to finally identify any level of illness in his body. Only in the last year has he identified his fibromyalgia. His general practitioner identified it, but he still can't get the VA to accept it as a diagnosis.

Rae H. I was raised in an environment of chaos. My father was an alcoholic, and my mother had serious emotional problems. I was the youngest of six children by eleven years, and by the time I was five years old all my siblings had moved out. My closest sister left under very traumatic circumstances, after the discovery of sexual abuse in the home. Interestingly, although a social worker documented my mother's emotional state and my sister's sexual abuse, I remained in the home. I will never understand why the state didn't intervene further. Although there was incest, I have believed throughout the years that the most damage was done by the sheer volume of chaos, by my mother's cold and withdrawn manner, and by the physically abusive molestation perpetrated upon me by a neighbor. When I went through therapy and experienced "body memories" from the neighbor's abuse, I understood the patterns of "holding" and "tightness" that my body had maintained throughout my entire life. Based on my personal and professional experiences, I do believe there is a correlation between the body's learned pattern of responding to stressors and the later eruption of fibromyalgia.

Cydney B. I believe that FM is probably the result of many traumas and stresses. I feel there may be some sort of either immune-system breakdown or adrenal fatigue or something else caused by sustained "fight-or-flight" reactions. My parents died when I was a teenager in the early 1960s. I knew of no one else who didn't have a father when my own father died of a heart attack at age forty-six. I was thirteen. My mother was an alcoholic and died two and a half years later. It was a child's worst nightmare come true. I lived in terror for another twenty-five years. I was running through life, just hoping nothing else would happen! In my late thirties, I started therapy, and these issues got worked out. But I feel all those years of terror did something to my body that caused FM to emerge.

Donnie M. I feel my FM was brought on by trauma and stress, beginning after my ovary removal and continuing through the surgical change of life. I was divorced at the time, alone, scared to death, supporting myself, and I had to work at a very stressful, thankless job. Things just continued to get worse for me, but I did marry my present husband during that period. Over the next four years, I had two major TMJ surgeries on both sides of my face, plus surgery on my nose for a deviated septum. All of this was done in an attempt to get rid of the horrid headaches I endured, but, instead, my health deteriorated.

After those three surgeries, the headaches got worse and I also had pain in my shoulders, neck, and back. I have known nothing but pain since my ovaries were removed. Since my early twenties I have suffered with headaches that have been diagnosed every way you can imagine. It was when the chronic fatigue hit that I got diagnosed with polymyalgia rheumatica (a progressive form of arthritis that causes pain and stiffness in the joints and muscles, as well as possible blindness).

I have often wondered if FM is inherited. I have many memories of my paternal grandmother walking around very slowly, unable to even sweep her floors and standing out by her well with a dipper of water, taking medications for her headaches. She was always sick, and no one ever said why.

Charlene M. I had three car accidents in five years. The first happened in 1995, when I was rear-ended. The second happened in 1996, when I was again rear-ended. The third happened in 1999, when I was broadsided. Through it all, the pain from the first accident continued.

I have heard that most people with FM have been abused. I was in two abusive marriages. I was first married in 1977. We began having trouble in 1978. He was physically abusive. We had a daughter in 1979, and he became more abusive, both physically and mentally. I divorced him in 1980. I got married again in 1981, and things were fine until I became pregnant in 1983. The marriage went downhill from there. He was mentally abusive. We had a son in 1984. We divorced in 1985.

Penny G. I think my illness is caused by a whole chain of traumatic events, starting with being sexually abused as a preteen, followed by struggles in my teens and twenties. I also am quite a perfectionist. I went back to school in my forties and worked full-time and took care of my family for four years, and that finally finished me off. I graduated in May 2000 and was diagnosed the next month with fibromyalgia. I also had a surprise pregnancy at forty, when my older children were twelve and fifteen. My youngest daughter is a total blessing to me, but the pregnancy and childbirth were very hard on my body.

Sondra H. I think there was a chain of events and traumas in my life that probably triggered FM. Within several years, I underwent a couple of significant surgeries, was involved in two automobile accidents, and underwent another surgery that resulted in chemical peritonitis, which really took its toll on me. It was almost fatal.

Nancy D. My job was becoming overwhelming; my workload grew big enough for two. It involved production typing, so specific in format that hiring a temporary worker was not an option. I typed at high speeds for seven to eight hours a day, with no breaks or lunches, for three to four months. My arms went numb, and I woke up many times during the night because of pain or numbness in my arms. Every morning I felt worse. Pretty soon it became exhausting just to put on simple makeup and comb my hair. It hurt to pull on pantyhose and to pull up the blankets in bed. I was developing symptoms of FM without realizing it. First the left forearm, elbow, and fingers went bad. When those symptoms were duplicated in the right arm, I called my doctor to ask for a referral to a neurologist. I was sure I had a pinched nerve. My doctor instead sent me to a rheumatologist, whose only available appointment was several weeks away. I waited, and kept calling for a possible earlier appointment. I typed on, each day doing more damage to myself. My sick leave was used up, but survival demanded that I keep going to work. It took a lot longer to get ready for work because of the worsening irritable bowel syndrome, the numb forearms and shaky fingers, and those darned pantyhose. Finally, the day came when I saw the rheumatologist. It was that doctor who sent me to a physical therapist, which saved the use of my arms and hands. By the next day, I was no longer working.

Six months later, I had an accident involving whiplash. The front of my shoe caught a ridge in the corner of the sidewalk, and I slid about five to seven feet until my right temple hit the side of a metal newspaper vending machine. Immediately a few angels showed up, including an off-duty fireman who stayed right there and kept me down and checked my vitals. An off-duty nurse was walking by and happened to have a cup of ice for a soda, which she applied to the cut above my eye. She also described the wound and what to expect. Angels somehow show up at the most needed times. Even so, however, things can go wrong. The fall caused lots of damage to the cervical area of my spine, chronic pain, and a degenerative spine condition.

FM was controversial at that time, so no doctor spoke of it in terms of a diagnosis. They spoke of it as "symptoms." A doctor explained that it was like the chicken-or-the-egg question: Legally, in terms of my worker's comp coverage, what came first is impossible to answer.

Rae H. I believe that FM is a body's response to trauma, either prolonged (e.g., childhood trauma) or acute (e.g., an accident). It is almost as if the body pulls in upon itself in a "clench" and then reacts to external stimuli. It is as though the body is in a chronic state of defense. I don't believe this could occur without some kind of precipitating trauma. And I believe there is a genetic predisposition toward a particular body's reacting to trauma in such a way as to create the chemistry that results in FM. In my own case, I had a fairly chaotic childhood, with a number of traumatic events. Additionally, I'd been in a number of rear-end collisions throughout the years and carried a lot of tension and stress in my body. But I believe the final trigger for the eruption of FM was the excessive and prolonged stress of graduate school in combination with full-time work, long commuting hours, and a stressful financial situation at home.

Gina H. I'd worked as a school crossing guard for eleven years when I fell off the curb and bruised my left side. I began having pain, but nobody knew why. I also fell down a flight of steps at my mother's house. Do I think these events caused my illness? I don't know. I just know I haven't been the same since they took place.

Lindamarie M. Many transitions have occurred in my path while living with FM, some positive and some very disruptive. The most terrifying ordeals before FM were the abuses I endured: gang rapes, rapes, child sexual abuse/rape/molestation, and much daily verbal and physical abuse. I am thirty-nine years old, and my first twenty-five years were filled with invasion and intrusion and horror that ripped my life apart. Many years of clinical therapy have helped me walk tall; however, the other invader that took control of my life was these health disorders, with FM being the instigator.

Cheryl W. My story begins when I became aware that I'd awakened every day since age twenty-one feeling like a Mack truck had run over me. Raised by two alcoholic parents, I later came to realize that I had suffered emotional, physical, and sexual abuse. In addition to being a mother and the caretaker of my family at a very young age, I played sports and exercised to survive. I learned to stay on the go, and I was constantly living in fight-or-flight mode. I put myself through college, taking a full load of classes, playing on the tennis team, and working twenty hours per week. I had four car accidents, none of which I was treated for; one major sports injury to my knee, requiring three surgeries; and a host of other minor injuries and accidents over the years.

I was diagnosed with endometriosis at age twenty-one, which caused immense pain and many trips to the ER. I had two other major surgeries besides the one on my knee. I spent most of my life working sixty to eighty hours per week running my own businesses, first as a tennis professional and then as a real estate broker. I gave up tennis due to the swelling in my knee from a botched operation, followed by inadequate and painful physical therapy. The swelling and pain were a daily event for fifteen years. I gave up my sixty-five-thousand-dollar-a-year real estate job at age thirty-nine because I was in too much pain.

▲▲▲

As you can see from these stories, trauma comes in many forms. All of it requires emotional healing. If you choose to talk about childhood physical or mental abuse, treat yourself gently. Get the support of your loved ones and a trained mental-health counselor. Don't do it alone. I made the decision to let go of my memories while working with an energy healer and my longtime counselor. I also relied on the love of my partner and on my friends, with whom I could talk about the pain. I believe the action I took peeled away another layer of the onion, a visual tool I use when I think of finding remission from fibromyalgia. We know FM is not a mental illness, and we know childhood abuse by itself doesn't cause fibromyalgia, but dealing with traumatic memories can go a long way in helping each of us begin to heal.

Everyday Solutions and Things That Really Work

This is a nuts-and-bolts chapter to help you live a better-quality life with FM. The women I interviewed offered lots of tips—methods they have developed over the years for living with a chronic, painful illness. People don't learn these things overnight. Helpful hints come as a result of thinking long and hard about adjusting to a new life, and after accepting the fact that you aren't physically the same as you once were. They come once you decide to take charge of your daily routine and your self-care in a proactive way, and once you decide to make the necessary changes that will allow you energy and time left over to enjoy yourself. The saying "Necessity is the mother of invention" translates for an FM'er into "Do everything you can to make your daily life easier."

Think of all the ways you have already changed your life to accommodate FM. By now you probably have proven to yourself that you can lower stress, take good care of yourself, and help your friends and family understand what you are up against. You may have come to recognize the difference between getting projects done in a healthy way and overdoing. This chapter can equip you with even more tools for living effectively with this illness. In it, the women tell us about the importance of getting regular rest, accepting their limits, making adjustments in their routines at home and at work, planning their day, and changing their diet. They also share creative responses to living with the pain, fatigue, and cognitive difficulties brought on by FM. The chapter's message is this: Use as many tips and tricks as you need to help you get through the day.

Here's another important point to consider: If necessary, reframe your thinking so that it doesn't feel like a loss to change your way of life to better cope with FM. All people—even those who never become chronically ill—experience big life transitions they didn't plan for. A strong person changes with the times.

GETTING ENOUGH REST

Rest periods throughout the day are very important to someone living with FM. At my house, we call it "having a rest." I go upstairs, sit in my chair by the bed, and read for a few minutes. For this purpose we have an old Morris chair that is covered with pillows and a small fleece blanket. Then it's nap time! Regular napping was new to me when I was first diagnosed. I learned the art of a good nap after my foot surgery. I would come home from work and sleep until dinnertime. Pain takes a lot out of you, and napping can recharge your batteries a bit so you can accomplish more during your day.

The bed is my sanctuary. I keep it outfitted with flannel sheets year-round and with the perfect old, flat pillow. My sister-in-law gave me a feather bed for my birthday, and it's heaven—four fluffy inches of softness that mutes the sharp pain in my elbows and hips. Buy the best bed you can afford to. Sleep is difficult for people with FM, so start at the ground up. A comfortable bed, bedding, and pillow are obvious needs, but also think of your entire sleeping area as a big part of the treatment of your illness. I have had a measure of success adjusting my sleeping area for optimum comfort. I prefer a dark room with lamps and a ceiling light with a dimmer. That way, there is enough light to read by, to find my medications, and to complete my bedtime rituals. Also, soft, soothing light to accompany meditation and music is so comforting.

The quietest area of your home should be where you sleep. Try to limit interruption and wake-ups by pets. This is called "good sleep hygiene," and it is of the utmost importance to those of us who have FM.

Sisu G. "Resting" does not mean sitting down. Talking on the telephone is not resting, and talking on the telephone while watching TV is even less restful. Promising yourself a nap later is a useless strategy. Do it now.

Keep your bedroom tidy. Seriously, you're going to spend a lot of time resting. Keep the area where you rest cheerful, calm, and comfortable. I had to buy new pillows. Get blankets and other things that make you comfortable and happy, because you're going to be seeing a lot of them.

Katie G. When I go to sleep, either at night or for a nap, I turn the phone ringer off. This ensures an uninterrupted sleep and a false sense that I am immune from the outside world, because my rest period is a sacred time to restore and recharge my body. I don't wash my hair or shower every day, and often I go outside (especially to work) without makeup. My apartment is not the immaculate living space I envision it to be, but if I need to sleep or rest, that takes precedence.

Rachel B. I know that a good night's sleep can help, and I also know that FM doesn't allow good, refreshing sleep. Taking the supplement melatonin helps me to get up to five hours of dreamless sleep, deep enough that I don't wake up every half hour. Listening to my favorite music keeps me relaxed until it's time to get up without staring at the clock every five minutes. It is also helpful to go to bed at the same time every night.

Diane H. Fatigue is caused by poor sleep, so a person with FM should also be tested for sleep apnea or other sleep disorders.

Jean T. Be good to yourself. If you are tired, don't push yourself. Try to rest. You will feel better. I love a hot shower, hot as I can stand it, especially on my back, shoulders, and head. It loosens muscles that I didn't know I had, except for the fact that I'm stiff and I hurt. A shower is a good thing to do before going to bed, and in addition I have a sheepskin topper on my mattress. Oh my! It's heaven, especially after that hot shower.

Rachel B. It's important to make sure you plan the day ahead and avoid too many activities that require physical activity. If a long activity is scheduled, make sure you get enough rest periods, and listen to your body. Do not overexhaust yourself.

SETTING LIMITS

Setting limits in any area has always been difficult for me. In my old life, I was always one of the last people to go home from work on a holiday. I would volunteer to work on Mother's Day or Thanksgiving if we had flowers left over. When friends asked for help, or even if they didn't ask, I would help them move, sell their cast-off items for extra money, or do any number of "helpful" things, beyond my body's limit.

After diagnosis, it took me many years to be able to say no, mean it, and not feel guilty. Once I learned how, I was amazed by how well it works! Just tell your friends, "Today I can't go shopping or help you, but maybe I can tomorrow." Limit your activities so that you get enough rest and can do the things that are important to you. If helping a friend is important and makes you happy, by all means do it. But realize your limits. If you can take an hour to help someone and still feel okay afterwards, you haven't pushed your limit.

Acceptance is a large part of setting limits. Before you can decide what your limits are, you have to understand and accept the fact that you have fibromyalgia. You have moved to a different phase of your life that includes rest as a part of your recovery. This was very hard for me. I had always been able to accomplish—all at one time—every task I set out to do. I had the energy to spend the day cleaning my gardens and applying bark. Now I know that tidying the gardens every day for a few minutes is the way to guarantee I will not overdo it and pay for it later. During the many months of working on this book, I made my priorities writing, resting, and seeing my doctors. I had to give up gardening, seeing my friends, and other interests. I had to set limits in order to be able to finish the project and enjoy it along the way.

Accepting that you can't do everything at once is a big accomplishment. It doesn't mean you have to miss out on life; it means you must rest more and set goals and limits. Deciding what is really important to you is paramount. Doesn't it seem like most people put themselves last on the list of what's important? Now, in order to recover, you must put your needs up close to the top.

Lalenya R. I have to limit my activities greatly. If I've slept, I must do most of what I can in the morning before fatigue and pain is exacerbated. I've stopped beating myself up for being unable to complete simple tasks or do what I used to do pre-FM.

Victoria M. Allow the body time out, and become aware of how much you can cope with. Stay within the boundaries of what is right for you, and when you're ready gradually push those boundaries a little at a time.

Cybill C. My tips for coping on a daily basis are to accept the fact that you cannot do it all. Lots of rest is needed. The world will not come to a crashing halt because the dishwasher wasn't emptied or because the kids had to eat cereal for dinner. You have to accept that with FM you give up a portion of control over your life. Don't push yourself or you will pay for it later.

Marcia D. I try to pace myself. I used to clean my whole house in a day, and now it takes me all week. It takes me one day to clean one room. By the time I get it done, it's time to start over. I used to vacuum every day. Now, if I get it done once a week, that's great. I've been trying to paint the house for over a year and it's still not done. So I just do what I think I can do. If I overdo it, I'm down for three or four days or a week or however long it takes to recover.

Cydney B. I set the kitchen timer for twenty minutes of activity at a time. Afterward I rest for a while before moving on to the next task. This was so hard for me to accept. But it had been suggested by books, my doctor, and my physical therapist so often, and I knew that my "cleaning frenzies"—as I called my usual cleaning style—were not working. But to force myself to sit down and do nothing for a half hour was just so hard. It felt like giving in. Then I finally did it when I had gotten to the point where I would spend a couple days in terrible pain and fatigue after a cleaning frenzy. And it worked so well. I lived to clean another time! Later that same day! Accepting limitations was the hardest and still is the hardest thing, because as time goes on there are more and more limitations. I am not any better now about accepting them than I was in the beginning, eight to ten years ago.

Kay B. Find out what you can and can't do. Don't do what you can't, and don't allow yourself to be nagged into going somewhere you don't want to go. I am my own best friend and worst enemy, and I have learned to recognize those attributes in myself. I don't allow myself to be pressured into action I know would be bad for me. On the other hand, if there is something I like to do—I love to shop at the Goodwill store—I save up the energy, and then I can do it.

ADJUSTING AT HOME AND AT WORK

I've always gone without a coat and hat. Even in Seattle I never carried an umbrella. After my diagnosis, I started paying attention to my body temperature and the difficulties in regulating it. Now I wear a hat every time I go out. Sometimes I even wear one inside in the early morning while I wait for my house to heat up. You lose a lot of heat from an uncovered head, and you might be surprised at how cozy a soft cotton-fleece hat feels. Find a few nice ones. You don't have to wear a stocking hat! Dress in layers of soft clothing. That way, it's easy to add and subtract clothes throughout the day. Bottom line: Do whatever it takes to stay warm. Cold weather affects FM. Women have told me their bodies are great barometers.

Taking time to look nice will boost your spirits. Don't feel invalidated by people who say, "But you look so good! You can't be sick." I will not conform to society's idea of what an ill person looks like. What *does* an ill person look like, anyway? I am just me. My approach to my personal appearance has become simpler. I still shower every morning to warm up my muscles, but my waist-length hair only gets washed every other day. Keeping comfortable with long hair takes a few tricks. I was discussing with a friend who has knee-length hair how painful it is to wear a ponytail, and she gave me a few tips. She suggested I use a loose braid to keep my hair out of the way during the day. Women with FM often have difficulty raising their arms for the time it takes to comb out long hair. If you have this problem, braid your hair before you go to bed at night; it takes less time to comb out the next morning. Another tip I follow is to use a chopstick or pick to hold my hair up in a roll. It looks nice and is quick to do.

Take time to organize your kitchen so that food preparation is easier. I cut up salad ingredients and place them in separate containers so I can make lunches and dinners quickly. I keep easy-to-prepare food and snacks available so there is always something avavilable to eat when I take my medications. Staying on top of things is equally important in my work area. I file constantly to avoid the stress of losing an important item.

Sisu G. My employers and coworkers know about my illness. My job description involves very few sick days, so I have to be there. On the worst days I wear hot packs under my clothing. I'm in rough shape in the mornings, so every weekend I line up a week's worth of outfits in my closet. I write myself a checklist every night to make sure I have keys, ID badge, etc.

Get a big terry-cloth bathrobe for when you're too tired to dry off from the bath. And an electric toothbrush is a wonderful invention for when you're at the end of the day and just want to collapse.

Put a tall chair in your kitchen to use when you're at the counter chopping food and doing other food prep.

Nancy D. I had to replace my wardrobe with loose cotton clothes, and I bought a down comforter because it is lightweight enough to tug on. I bought lots of lightweight plasticware for the kitchen. Four years ago I couldn't find plastic plates anywhere, so I went to a Chinese restaurant-supply store, where I got some great lightweight dishes.

Jean T.   One of my best coping strategies is in my kitchen. Because of my pain and lack of balance, I had an awful time preparing meals. It took so much effort that I found myself eating too much fast food. Now I can hardly stand the thought of a hamburger. Besides, they are not good for you, and the habit is too expensive. I have started buying quite a lot of precooked, frozen food from the Schwan's man, who makes deliveries of prepared foods in his freezer truck (see Resources). I spent quite a while selecting items that are to my liking. I find that it isn't any more expensive than buying regular groceries, because you don't have the spoilage. Now I only buy staples from the grocery store.

Don't ever stand if you can find a way to sit. You must conserve your strength for more important things. I bought an office chair with five wheels that I use in the kitchen. I pull myself around using the edges of the cupboards. The seat is a little lower than I would like, but I can manage until I figure out how to keep the pneumatic adjustment from going lower.

If you have small children, you must let them do as much for themselves as possible. It's not selfish to expect this of them. They will need other kinds of help from you in doing things that they can't do for themselves. It doesn't hurt a child to learn how to vacuum the high-traffic areas, pick up and put things away, put the dishes in the dishwasher, or take the trash out. I have taught Austin, my grandson, how to swipe the debit card and fill the car with gas. It makes him feel so grown up.

It is so hard to manage even though I live by myself. It must be really overwhelming for someone with a family.

Lindamarie M.   I use a stool at the sink to help me keep my balance and decrease pain. It's also important to use appropriate tools for writing, cooking, and reading. When doing laundry, I ask for help from my family members. I make sure to keep baskets at hip or waist level so I don't have to do so much bending, which tires me easily.

PLANNING YOUR DAY, YOUR WEEK, YOUR LIFE

In the beginning of my illness, I quickly realized that a single activity, such as a doctor's appointment, was the only thing I could schedule in a day. Getting up and getting ready to leave, driving to the appointment, seeing the doctor, and driving home sometimes is all I can do for that day. Planning more than one activity away from home is still hard. It always takes more time than I think it will. A visit with friends or family or seeing a movie is still considered the day's one event.

Try using a calendar or a chalkboard to help you plan your week more easily. I write down each appointment, call, or trip, no matter how small, on my calendar. This helps me to think ahead about my day and week. As long as they're planned for, I can easily include a few "easy" tasks like "just stopping here for a minute" or going food shopping without taking special care to conserve energy. Sometimes I miss my spontaneity, but if I keep to a schedule I'll have a little extra energy to do a fun activity or two during the week.

I tend to have a better day—meaning less pain and fatigue—if I stagger my tasks into two categories, mental and physical. It seems to take less of my precious energy to finish a household chore (physical), rest, and then balance my checkbook, make a phone call, or send an e-mail (mental). Avoiding crowding too many physical tasks into a day reserves more energy.

Kay B. I measure my energy. I gauge my tasks by the amount of energy they require and by the pain I'm in when I wake up in the morning. I do something every day. I do not allow myself to be a bump on the recliner, although I give myself permission to veg out some days. I do things I enjoy and can accomplish sitting down. I ask for help from my husband when I need it. I don't wait till he asks if I need help. Our relationship is quite sound, which I think is in part because of my illness.

Katie G. Every day I make lists of what to do. Of course, there are multiple lists! It does seem to help me stay more organized, and it gives me a sense of accomplishment and a road map for strategizing my day.

Sisu G.   The only way to have a social life is to schedule carefully in advance. Allow time to rest and recover. I actually started updating people by e-mail, which has proved a great way to keep everyone educated. I lost half my friends to this illness, because I can't go and do the things I used to, but I've learned that the remaining friends are stronger and truer than I ever could have expected. So I set up a website for my close friends, and only they have access to it.

Lindamarie M.   I make sure to space out the events on my calendar. I reserve my energy for doctor's appointments and errands. Keeping in mind the schedule for the following day, I rest as much as I need.

CREATIVE RESPONSES TO LIVING WITH THE SYMPTOMS

Tips for Dealing with Pain and Fatigue

The hardest lesson FM taught me was to set limits and pace myself. But it's imperative to do so, because once the pain gets out of control it is hard to reign back in. At those very difficult times, I meditate, using the same guided imagery I have followed for years. I have found that using a meditation tape with headphones is a great way to get started. If you haven't meditated before, it helps to hear a soft, slow voice in your ear. It drowns out the thoughts of everyday life and seems to help the images come easier. I use a chakra-clearing tape, among others. Tapes are available in metaphysical bookstores or spiritual stores. Or try a meditation group. Self-hypnosis or hypnosis done by a professional may help with pain. At other times, I ride out the flare with diversions such as writing poetry or reading. Our correspondents offer additional suggestions below:

Mary H.-B. Biofeedback is great for dealing with stress. Yoga is great for learning to center yourself. Massage therapy is great for relaxing. For fatigue, take time out each day for a nap.

Denise P. I rest a lot while I'm at home since it is hard to do very much physical labor. To help with the pain, I have taken classes on self-hypnosis and on self-massage for pressure points in the feet. These methods don't always help, but it is better than taking pain pills all the time. A short nap really helps to relieve fatigue, even if it is just putting my head on my desk at lunchtime.

Cybill C. I stretch every night, and that really helps with the pain. Sometimes if the pain is intense, I use Ben-Gay, but I try to avoid using it often because it hurts my skin.

Val T. I use a hot tub. Additionally, my doctor's own recipe for ointment relieves pain far better than anything you can buy over the counter. I limit myself and my activities as needed; I take saunas, get massages, and stretch all the muscle groups gently, usually in the mornings when I am very stiff. I take supplements, including malic acid and magnesium, grape-seed extract, multivitamins, vitamins E and C, and glucosamine chondroitin, which my doctor just recommended for my degenerative disk disease.

Nancy D. Hot baths are wonderful; I am lucky to have an oval tub so I can maneuver around and get out of it in a few different ways. My arms are shot after a shower, so I try to bathe every couple of days. Massage always helps but is not affordable. One therapy that intrigues me is stone massage, which basically involves placing flat, round rocks that have been either heated or chilled against painful parts of the body. I keep some river rocks in the freezer for this purpose. A therapist who does this for sixty-five dollars an hour told me on the phone to use warm rocks heated in a pan of hot water on all the places that hurt and then to put cold rocks on the same places. This therapy is difficult to do alone, but I have woken up on many mornings with a warm rock under my neck that started out frozen the night before.

Rae H. I start the day with a hot shower, during which I do energy work and prayer work. It makes all the difference. I journal and write poetry; I can't imagine life without these gifts of expression.

My spirituality is very important. When I go to my "sanctuary" in my heart, I feel physically better, emotionally better, and I see life just a little brighter than it was when I was in the cave of despair. Walking on the treadmill, no matter how bad I feel, is a true gift. I never step off regretting that I took the time to exercise. I listen to music, especially when treadmilling, and bring that energy into my heart. I watch funny movies to make sure that I laugh. And I always remember to appreciate my blessings. As horrible as I feel, as frightened as I get, I can measure many more things to be grateful about than to lament.

▲▲▲

Tips for Dealing with "Fibro Fog"

Maybe you recognize this scene: You are in a big department store, such as Target or Home Depot. There are lots of people and colorful items. It's a bright and loud store with children running around and shoppers and their carts vying for space in the aisles. Suddenly you have no idea what it is you have come to purchase. Or worse, everything catches your eye and you begin to fill a cart with stuff you don't need. This has happened to me many, many times. I have learned to shop in off-peak hours when I am at my freshest. I avoid the chemical and pesticide aisles, both the lawn and garden and the home-cleaning sections. I take a list. I make my purchases and get out.

Such is a typical episode of "fibro fog" or "FM brain fog," characterized by difficulties processing, understanding, and retaining information. Many of the tips shared in the earlier section on planning, such as writing every scheduled event on a calendar, can help you to keep your life straight in the face of this frustrating symptom.

I couldn't survive without a list. I've been a listmaker all of my life, but now if I forget to write things down, I am sunk. This includes obvious things like, "Go to bank; take deposit," or "Go to post office; take mail." And the Post-Its I go through! I always put them in two places: on the mirror and by the front door. They list the most urgent items that need to be attended to, such as "Bosco is at the beauty salon." No, it's not enough to miss seeing my dog around. After four hours, it requires a note.

Here's a description of how I managed to write this book. My brain doesn't work like it once did, so I had to come up with creative ways to accomplish this lengthy and fairly complex task. In essence, I went about it the old-fashioned way. I wrote in longhand, and I utilized the help of a typist and editor. Typing for any length of time is difficult, and I am slow at it. And because it is hard for me to remember what I can't see, I don't use a computer for writing. I work on a slant board so I have less neck strain. I taped the pages from each chapter on the wall, which helped me to understand the order of the subchapters. I used two copies for making changes: one to read, and one to make notes on.

The energy required for work of any kind is a huge commitment for someone with chronic pain. I am unable to work at even a minimal part-time job, but writing is doable as long as I can move around, take many breaks, and pace myself. Writing this book took me many months, an hour at a time.

If work is part of your life, you already know what it takes to get yourself up and out of the house every day. It is a lesson in organization. Do everything you can to cut down on stress. Stress is a huge culprit in the intensity of my episodes of fibro fog. Plan ahead, and be organized. Remember, perfection isn't possible, and who wants it anyway? Be easy on yourself, and take time to rest and relax every day.

Driving is the hardest thing I do. Seattle is rated fourth in the nation for the noise, the fumes, and the amount of single-minded concentration a driver needs to get from point A to point B. I learned about the September 11 tragedy while driving to my therapist's office. Like all Americans, I felt shock, fear, confusion, anger, and sadness throughout my whole body. I have driven to my therapist's many times, and I always follow the same route. It takes about twenty-five minutes to get there. But on September 11, I was forty-five minutes late because I got lost.

Those were extenuating circumstances. Most days, it works well simply to allow myself plenty of time to get wherever I need to go. Being late causes stress that I just don't need. When planning an event out of the house, allow more time in your schedule than you think you'll need for traffic and last-minute preparation.

The first time I got lost driving in my city, I was afraid. Exits I had passed every day didn't look familiar, and I couldn't find a landmark. Now I know these breaks in memory will pass, and suddenly I will recognize where I am. It's as though everyday life slips into a time warp, and then a few minutes later I am back in real time.

Jean T. The Alpha Stim 100 (a microcurrent unit) clears up what I call brain fog, which makes you feel like your head is so thick you have trouble functioning, and it seems like everything happens in slow motion. Before I began using the Alpha Stim, sometimes the brain fog would not clear up for a whole day.

Gina H. When I go to the doctor, I follow the same route every time so I won't get lost. I write in my journal what medication I have taken so I won't take it again. I keep a list of people who have called me so I can remember to call them back.

DIET

People will do anything to get better—right? But when it comes right down to it, are they willing to change their diet?

It is so hard to leave behind comfort food when you are feeling bad and want the soothing emotions that a plate of chicken and dumplings can bring. Unfortunately, when we feel the worst—in pain and exhausted—we often lack the energy to cook well for ourselves. But even I, a dedicated Powerbar and Pepsi woman (and that's for breakfast!), must admit that diet plays a huge role in feeling better if you have FM. The healthier your diet, the healthier you will be overall—and that goes double for those of us with a chronic illness.

There are so many diet suggestions out there, it can make your head spin. I've found my own. Consuming smaller, more frequent meals containing some type of protein has really helped to boost my energy levels. I take chromium picolinate once daily to stabilize my carbohydrate metabolism so I don't undergo a big drop in blood sugar between meals. This has also helped tremendously. Before adding the supplement, my pain level would skyrocket between meals and I would feel very tired.

Metabolism of carbohydrates seems to benefit from consuming them in combination with other foods, so I try to eat my carbohydrate snack, such as a Powerbar or cereal, with dinner. Try to take your medication with food; that way your stomach lining will be less affected over the long term. Also, I've noticed that my pain meds actually give more relief if taken with food. A fairly substantial mini-meal works the best, not just a bite. Try to keep snacks available so that when you're hungry, when it's time to take your medication, or when you're feeling low in energy you can easily go to the kitchen and grab something. We keep Powerbars, granola bars, apples, and cheese on hand. A chunk of Asiago cheese and a cut-up apple makes the perfect between-meal pick-me-up.

I build my daily meals around chicken or fish and salads and vegetables. Maintaining a good balance of protein, vegetables, fruits, carbs, and fats suits me and my family; that way I never feel like I have given up something or am missing out. Undoubtedly, however, other FM'ers find that a more restrictive diet proves vital to managing their symptoms. Below, a few of the women share what works for them. Don't be worried by the fact that some of the eating plans they've adopted contradict one another. Food is like religion: There's no one right plan for everyone. What should you do in the face of so many apparently conflicting suggestions about diet? Inform yourself, to be sure, but then learn to trust your own body and to pay attention to the subtle signs it sends you.

Katie G. Diet has been very important. I have eliminated caffeine, alcohol, sugar, refined and processed foods, dairy products, and wheat. My abdomen no longer swells as it did after eating wheat and glutens, and my GI tract is great; it gives me no problems. This is basically the diet we are all told about: veggies, fruits, lean meats, nuts, brown rice. Such a change in diet takes a little adjustment, but it is well worth it. Eating often and nutritiously cannot be overstated. I eat three to four times a day, sometimes every few hours. Drinking lots of water is also important.

Patricia S. By accident, I found that the nightshade vegetables (tomatoes, bell peppers, zucchini, squash, eggplant) increase pain for me. I didn't believe it when I first heard it suggested, so I said, "Prove this!" I cooked myself up a big frying pan of peppers and tomatoes and ate it, and I was absolutely in wretched tears the next day. It took four days for my pain to go back to baseline. Besides the nightshade family, many other fruits and vegetables stir up my pain, including apples, bananas, and melons. Peaches are one of the few fruits I can eat. A lot of women say that berries cause more pain. Berries are known to be very irritating to the bladder, so the women affected may suffer bladder-related symptoms. On the other hand, some people are absolutely unaffected by fruits and vegetables. That's why I believe this disease is not one entity, it manifests somewhat differently in everybody. Some of it is triggered by derangement in chemical neurotransmission, and everybody's chemistry is different.

I also find that heavily spiced foods trigger more pain. Meat doesn't affect me; I eat a lot of meat. I went to one of those health spas where they serve raw vegetables, and the pain had me howling at the moon. I changed my diet to heavily cooked meats and grains and dairy products. I don't drink coffee; I gave up all caffeine. I gave up soda; I gave up Nutrasweet. Certain other foods I no longer eat as often, simply because you hear people saying they're no good for you. For example, I'm lighter on wheat than I used to be. I was a big bread eater.

Women with FM should be very careful with their diet, including avoiding getting hungry; hunger can lead to problems with hypoglycemia. I don't know if I'm actually hypoglycemic, but when I get hungry, I get very weak and my pain actually increases. When I am really hungry, I start to feel more achy all over, and I don't recoup immediately after eating. I've screwed myself for the day, and I have to start all over again the next day. I now realize that I can't ignore my hunger. I can't say, "But I want to lose a couple of pounds." I need to keep my weight regular. I have to walk a thinner line. I've really cleaned up my life. That's not to say I don't enjoy any fun foods, but I'm careful about what my fun foods are.

Sisu G. Celiac disease is a genetic intolerance to gluten. It causes the immune system to get all fired up, thinking that gluten is an attacker. The disease can be triggered at any point in your life, or you can be born with the gene already active, as with diabetes. When it's active, you get all kinds of autoimmune symptoms that may go away after you start eliminating gluten-containing foods from the diet. Sometimes it triggers other conditions such as lupus, MS, or epilepsy.

People are routinely tested for celiac disease in certain countries, for example Italy and Ireland. Here, it's more difficult to get a diagnosis. Screening is as simple as a blood test and an endoscopy. Anyone who has FM symptoms should be screened for celiac, because those who do have it may be able to vastly improve their condition by simply making a change in their diet. I got tested for celiac disease because my sister tested positive. My mother also has it. Now we're gluten-free. I'm better than I was. I still have FM, but I can do a great deal more, and I'm a thousand times healthier.

▲▲▲

Sisu makes a great point about celiac sprue, or gluten intolerance. If you do not test positive for celiac, yet you still feel you are sensitive to gluten or other food substances, have your doctor recommend a nutritionist. You can easily be tested, or test yourself, for food allergies by following a rotation diet. Identifying and correcting a food allergy or intolerance may make a dramatic difference in your illness. A book I recommend is *Optimal Wellness*, by Ralph Golan, M.D., which contains a substantial section on diet and food allergies. (See the comments of Dr. Jenefer Scripps Huntoon, in Chapter 12, for a naturopathic physician's take on diet and FM.)

DIVERSIONS

The women who responded to my survey reported employing many different diversions, small things that seem to help their day go a little better. For me, regular "visits" with my pets and walks in my gardens serve as momentary distractions from pain and fatigue. My exercise routine (see Chapter 5) helps, as do nocturnal walks. I take these walks for exercise, of course, but really I like to see inside people's homes! Imagining their lives, so different from each other's and from mine, takes my mind off the pain for a little while.

A diversion may be as simple as talking to a friend who has FM. It may be going to your computer and connecting in a chat room with other FM patients from all over the country. Reading is a good one, as is watching a video. Anything to take your mind off the pain and help you relax is a great diversion. After I take my first medication of the day, I sit in my rocker by the heater vent and read some sort of fiction (not a medical book!) for a half hour or so. This is my time to wake up a little and to let the medication go to work. I do it several times a day.

Marcia D. I like to do creative things, such as needlepoint, but I have limited use of my hands. My mom gave me some quilts that belonged to my aunt. They all need to be resewn by hand, and I have been trying to work on that, but I do three or four squares per night and I have to stop because my hands hurt. I like to garden, but it's a challenge to get down on my hands and knees to pull the weeds.

When we go to our home in eastern Oregon, it's like traveling back fifty years in time. It's very relaxing. I enjoy going up there. I even go and stay by myself for a week at a time. It takes away your everyday stress when it's just you to worry about and not the washing, the cleaning, the shopping, the paying of bills. I try to do that two or three times a year.

Denise P. Even on the days when the pain is bad, I make myself get up, get dressed, and go to work. On my days off I try to do something, even if it is just washing a few dishes, making the bed, or paying bills—anything to take my mind off the pain. What keeps me going is probably my grandson. He is so precious; I love him so much. I want him around me. Even though it is hard I try to keep him overnight at least once a weekend.

Cybill C.   I'm involved in a few different creative hobbies. I research a variety of topics on the Internet, and I write poetry. I like to put on music and dance with the kids.

Donna F.   I love to bake and try new recipes. I love to watch and hear my children play. I love to garden. My husband and I spend a lot of precious time alone together. All of these things I do for myself beyond treating FM. What drives me every day are my priorities, joys, and rewards all rolled into one. They are my spiritual life, my dear husband and children, my extended family, and all the pleasant joys life has to offer to a blessed stay-at-home wife and mother.

Katie G.   I love baseball. During baseball season my day can revolve around when the game is on. Walking and being outside always make me feel better. I love to walk around town and window shop or stop in the stores and say hello to people I know. I also love to putter in my apartment, reorganize, clean things out, etc. I swim sometimes, and I enjoy my volunteer work at the hospital and serving on the board. Being involved and helping, giving something of myself to others, makes me feel productive and worthwhile.

Walking has helped me tremendously, both to relieve stress and mental worry, and also to build endurance and strength. I find that alternating between walking, doing my exercises, cleaning my apartment, grocery shopping, and resting helps to restore my energy levels and keeps me balanced throughout the day. It was a little difficult at first to allow myself the rest I need, because I was so brainwashed by society that only weak or lazy people need to rest or to sleep (a few times) during the day. Now I see the tremendous benefits for the long-term. I feel smart when I pace myself and can recharge my batteries.

As you can see from these women's comments, diversions come in many forms. They include any "time out" taken for yourself and any behaviors or little rituals that bring an escape from the pain. Try including a few in your day.

SUMMARY: HELPFUL HINTS FOR LIVING WITH FM

Here is a convenient summary of some of the pointers given in this chapter:

Resting

◂ Learn the art of a good daytime nap

◂ Remember that resting doesn't mean talking on the phone or watching a stimulating TV show

◂ Practice good "sleep hygiene": Limit intrusions from pets and kids, keep the room as dark as possible while you're resting, and purchase the most comfortable and functional mattress, linens, and accessories you can afford

◂ Consider getting tested for sleep disorders such as sleep apnea

◂ Try a hot shower or bath before bedtime

◂ Go to bed at the same time every night

Setting Limits

◂ Practice the skill of saying "no"

◂ Learn to accept the limitations brought on by your illness. Let go of feeling like you need to "do it all"

◂ Put yourself and your health at the top of your list of priorities

◄ Learn—and honor—your own boundaries regarding what you can and can't do

◄ Set a timer to allow twenty minutes for an activity. When the timer goes off, stop what you're doing and rest for twenty or thirty minutes. The task will still be there after your rest period

Adjusting at Home and at Work

◄ Stay warm by wearing hats and dressing in layers

◄ Buy comfortable, loose-fitting clothes

◄ Wear hot packs under your clothing

◄ Simplify your approach to grooming (but remember that looking nice can boost your spirits!)

◄ If you work outside the home, select a week's worth of outfits on Sunday, prepare your lunch the night before, and post a checklist next to the door of things you need to take with you every morning (keys, ID badge, lunch, bus pass)

◄ Organize your kitchen to make food prep easier: Cut up salad ingredients ahead of time; keep nutritious snacks readily available; place a tall chair or stool next to the kitchen counter so you can sit while you're chopping; and purchase lightweight, plastic dishes and storage containers

◄ Consider signing up for delivery of prepared, frozen meals, if such a service is available in your area

◄ Conserve energy by sitting whenever you can. Use a rolling chair to wheel yourself around the kitchen, office, or utility room

◄ Let your kids and spouse help with housework

Planning Your Schedule

◀ Hang a poster-size calendar or whiteboard in a visible place, and write on it every appointment, errand, and phone call

◀ "Stagger" your tasks into two categories—mental and physical—and avoid crowding too many physical tasks into a single day or week

◀ This one bears repeating: Pace yourself! Avoid overdoing by carefully gauging your energy levels, setting limits, and sticking to them

Dealing with Pain and Fatigue

◀ Use meditation or guided imagery. To learn these skills, listen to audiotapes, join a meditation group, or go to a hypnotherapist

◀ Try biofeedback

◀ Stretch daily and engage in other forms of gentle exercise

◀ Get a massage

◀ Soak in a hot tub or take a hot shower or bath

Dealing with "Fibro Fog"

◀ Make lists, even of the smallest things you need to accomplish

◀ Stick Post-It notes everywhere: on the bathroom mirror, next to the kitchen sink, and on the front door

◀ Do everything possible to reduce stress, which is a major culprit in episodes of brain fog. Especially allow extra time for traffic and last-minute preparation

◀ Write down what medications and supplements you've taken and when. That way, you won't wonder, "Have I or haven't I?"

Diet

◀ Don't be overwhelmed by all the conflicting dietary advice that's available. Educate yourself about the basics of good nutrition, and then listen to your body and follow the subtle signs it sends you

◀ Consider getting tested (or testing yourself, through a rotation diet) for food intolerances or allergies

◀ Work with a nutritionist who's familiar with FM to develop an eating plan that's right for you

Diversions

◀ Several times a day, take a few minutes to do things you enjoy and that help you feel better, such as sitting or walking in your garden, spending time with your pets, or reading fiction

◀ Find a creative outlet: Write poetry, keep a journal, make art, or do needlepoint

◀ Watch a sport you love on TV

◀ Escape obligations for a few days by taking a vacation alone

CHAPTER

8

Dealing with the People Closest to Us

Living with fibromyalgia brings with it some inevitable challenges in our relationships with family, friends, and intimate partners. Sisu describes these issues:

> **Sisu G.** Illness places a tremendous burden on relationships—all relationships. And not merely because it involves chronic pain, physical challenges, a massive amount of adaptation, and a whole mess of medical information. No, this issue runs even deeper than that.
>
> When one person stays healthy and the other suddenly becomes chronically, seriously ill, it can be very damaging to a relationship. FM is not a shared experience. It happens internally. It doesn't show on the outside, so we have to educate anyone who would hope to understand. It challenges our ability to communicate those elements most fundamental to a relationship: our fears, our feelings, and our sense of self. This goes for the healthy person in the relationship, too. And without good communication, things don't work even under perfect conditions. Under the added pressure of chronic illness, things are even less likely to work when something big hits. Friendships are no different from love affairs in this regard. An injured or ill person will sometimes have trouble relating to the healthy world. A healthy person may find it difficult to relate to someone who is obviously experiencing something so personal and intense.

▲▲▲

SEEKING UNDERSTANDING AND ACCEPTANCE

To those of us who have fibromyalgia, the dichotomy it presents is obvious: We look great but feel awful. Many women tell me that their friends and family members refuse to believe in their illness. Some even doubt the existence of FM. This invalidation is almost as painful as the illness itself. We want so much to have the understanding and support of our loved ones, and when it is denied we feel angry and alone.

Gerry L. Fibromyalgia is invisible. We look good; we look normal. We are not bleeding or limping. We don't have swollen and deformed joints. The scars are inside. That's why it is so hard for some to believe in its existence. We can perform normally one day and the next cannot function at all.

A change took place when I said to a family member, "If my pain were categorized as malignant versus nonmalignant, you would have a whole different understanding of my condition, wouldn't you?"

Sisu G. It's tough, because people want you to be normal. My stepfather says I look so healthy, I can't possibly be sick. I don't always feel understood. Having FM is a very individual experience. The only way to understand it is to go through it, and I wouldn't wish that on anybody.

Donnie M. Do I feel understood? No way. I feel accepted as long as I don't talk about my medical problems and as long as I try to pretend I am not in pain. In other words, I have to be a darn good actress, not the real me.

Donna P. That is the biggest trouble with FM—you look great, so people think you are okay. When I was first diagnosed and had to quit my job, my employers could not understand. They begged me to stay, but there was no way I could continue to work.

Donna F. It's hard for family and friends to remember that I have physical limitations because of this condition. FM is clothed in the disguise of a clean, made-up exterior, because none of us want to look ill.

Gina H. Do I feel understood and accepted? No. I don't think any of us really feel understood unless we're talking to someone who's also going through it. Do I feel accepted? No, not really, unless the other person is feeling my pain. I don't think the millions of us who have FM will ever feel understood or accepted until the doctors can say with certainty what this disease can and will do.

Cydney B. I am not sure if I feel understood. I am not sure anyone who doesn't have FM can understand.

HEARING FROM FAMILY MEMBERS OF FM PATIENTS

To help us comprehend why those closest to us may have a hard time giving us the unconditional understanding and support we desire, let's consider their situation for a moment. Life partners and other family members of patients with chronic illness have a tough row to hoe. They, too, are likely to experience grief over what they and their family have lost with the onset of their loved one's condition, and they, too, may undergo a dramatic restriction in lifestyle as a result of the illness. In particular, family members of FM patients, just like the patients themselves, often must endure a frustrating lack of understanding from the outside world, including from other family members. Donna S.'s husband has fibromyalgia. Below, she writes of the difficulty of taking care of her husband without the support of their families:

Donna S. I felt confused when Don was diagnosed, because at the time I had no clue about what FM even was, and there was no information about it. I asked questions and received half answers. I was frustrated that the doctors couldn't tell us why my husband got it, and frustrated that there was no cure. The first year was filled with trying antidepressants, muscle relaxants, this drug, that drug. I felt like a pharmacist and still do. He is on so much medicine it makes my head spin at times.

We don't have the social life we used to. We did things with the kids, went to parks, went to the mall, rode four-wheelers, went camping. After my husband was diagnosed, however, we kept to ourselves because no one understands this condition or wants to learn about it. I won't sit with people and continue to defend why he doesn't work, or why his doctor doesn't just give him a pill. Camping is out now; Don is unable to sleep outside. We do a little camping in our backyard, but we used to have friends and family to share it with. Now that it's just us, it's not any fun.

I go to work and come home. I don't really go anywhere without taking my husband with me. I know how it feels to be cooped up in a house all day long with no one to talk to. It is very depressing for him. So I feel guilty if I go anywhere without him. I get very mad at times when others are going to parties or other recreational events and I am at home. I get mad when family members treat us like we have the plague and say things to me like, "Why do you stay with him?" Or, "There is nothing wrong with him; you're just letting him stay home and be lazy." Yet they don't take the time to call and say "Hi." I also get mad that Don sometimes doesn't trust me, that he is afraid I will leave him or send him away.

I am afraid he will attempt suicide again and I won't be there to stop him. I am afraid that no matter how many hours I work we are not going to have enough money to eat or pay the rent. At times I am afraid to go to work because I don't want to leave him alone; I never know from one hour to the next what could happen. I feel guilty that I can go to work and he can't. I see the pain he suffers as a man unable to support his family. I try to let him know that what he does for me at home is just as important, but no matter what I say it is just not enough. ·

I resent that when Don attempted suicide, his family made it out to be my fault over an argument. They didn't understand that it was because he didn't want to be a burden anymore. I resent that since the suicide attempt he is afraid to tell me anything for fear I will send him back to the psychiatric ward.

I resent that our family doesn't support us. Both of our families only hear what they want to hear. Don's family does not really understand what FM is and doesn't want to learn. They make comments like, "He only has a backache. Go get a shot or something. You have a bad doctor. You need a lawyer." They avoid him since the suicide attempt. This makes me very mad. He has had two surgeries, and his brother never called to see how he was doing. Nor was his family any kind of support to the kids and me when he attempted suicide. The only comment I got was, "You did the right thing, you got him help." What he went through at the hospital was not help; it was torture.

Even though we do not live far apart from each other, my family has never been close. We speak only occasionally. My sister is a nurse, and when I can't find the answer to a medical question or when I have a medical concern, I call her.

Sometimes I feel like I have no one to talk to. My friends don't understand his illness, and if I try to explain it, they change the subject. Don and I talk, but it's either about what kind of pain he is in today, or should we try this or that medication, or what we will tell the doctor next visit. My feelings, thoughts, and what I did at work are lost because my life revolves around him and FM.

I feel depressed because I have no one to lean on when things are really bad. Sometimes it is my own fault because I try to deal with everything myself and forget to ask for help. But I don't ask because I don't want to burden anyone with my problems. I have one friend in town who has been there for me when things get really bad. She has kept our son at her house and gets him to and from school. But she has her own family, and I try not to dump on her unless there is no other choice. We live in a small town. The nearest big city is about fifty miles away. To find a support group that deals with FM would be hard because I would have to drive miles to meetings.

We have two children, an eighteen-year-old daughter (mine before meeting Don), who is in the Army, and a ten-year-old son (Don's and mine). Kayla is trying to deal with this even though she is in Arizona. Leaving for the Army was a very hard decision for her, because at the time Don was in the hospital following his suicide attempt. But I told her there was nothing she could do here, and she needed to go and see what the real world was like. She got to talk to Don on the phone before she left, and the two of them made a pact that she would make it through basic training and he would get out of the hospital. Cody, our son, is a very active child. He loves basketball, Pokemon, and electronic games. He understands his dad's illness and knows when he needs to help him out. He gets upset at times if we plan something and Dad's just not up to doing it when the time comes. It is sometimes hard on him, but he has grown up with his dad having this and really knows no other way.

Meeting and talking with my friend Paula, a Reiki master, about finding spiritual peace was positive. She also has fibromyalgia and regularly gets updated information from the Internet. She has been a great deal of help in the last year. I keep reading and searching for answers on how to alleviate the pain Don suffers. I've learned to take things one day at a time and to make each day count. I read as much as I can find on FM—doing so helps. I feel the more I read and learn, the more I understand and can cope with it.

My faith in God has become stronger, and it is what keeps me going. I put all problems and concerns in His hand and go on. If I dwelled on everything that goes wrong around here, I would be in a padded cell somewhere.

Besides the inevitable loss experienced by family members of FM'ers, sometimes watching a chronically ill loved one deal doggedly with the challenges of her condition can inspire admiration, as Laura, Rachel B.'s partner, writes:

Laura I think Rachel has a tremendous amount of strength and determination. I have seen firsthand how much pain she is in at times, and how hard this is for her to bear. She continues to persevere, and she pushes herself to remain as independent and active as she can possibly be. She has tremendous inner strength and drive—you might even say she has a self-challenging spirit—which seem to keep her going long beyond what I or many others would even attempt.

She used to be a mountain climber, and I frequently think of the challenges she faces with FM as her Mt. Everest. She has had to depend on that same determination, drive, and sheer courage to get over the "mountain" presented by FM. I know the illness has taken a tremendous toll on her, physically and mentally, but I believe she will get through it and will someday stand on the summit of that mountain and celebrate. I look forward to that day. I will climb that mountain—by her side, every inch of the way—and join her in her celebration.

▲▲▲

SPOUSES AND PARTNERS

It is heartbreaking when your spouse or intimate partner cannot come to terms with the fact that you have a chronic illness. With the onset of FM, both your lives have been completely altered, and your husband may be feeling frustrated because there isn't anything he can do to help you. These are hard times. Your body has changed, your role in the family may have changed, and you lack the comfort of your life partner.

It was eye-opening for my partner to meet other people with FM. Before, when she knew only me with all of my symptoms and with the pain such a huge part of our lives, it seemed overwhelming, unbelievable. Maybe like yours, my partner was devastated when we found out FM could not be cured. Somehow, it helped to get to know others who battled FM; doing so made the illness more real. From there, I was able to show my partner that together we could live well, even though I have fibromyalgia.

Here's what other women have to say about FM's effects on their marriages:

Val T. I was terrified that my husband would no longer want to stay with me now that I was ill and hurt so badly. I couldn't keep up, and I couldn't always go out with him to socialize or do other activities. I was so afraid he would walk away. In the books I read on FM, there were many stories of husbands walking away from their wives after they were diagnosed.

Mea C. My spouse and I have drifted apart. He does his thing; I do mine. There's less sex, less laughter. He probably feels overwhelmed, but he keeps things to himself, so I don't know for sure. He doesn't want all the responsibility that has been thrust upon him, but that's too bad. I don't want FM.

Gina H. Let me start by telling you about the love of my life, my best friend, my husband. My husband was the man who would do anything for me and give me anything I wanted or needed. When I had a hysterectomy and they hit my bladder during surgery, I had to wear a catheter in the morning and at night. I was scared and angry about having to wear that thing. My husband took off work for six weeks to be there for me. He was the one who changed my catheter every day until it was removed. Even though it was on my body I could not bring myself to touch it. My husband was the man who cleaned my ears when I got my ears pierced, because I couldn't do that either. I wanted contacts because I'd been wearing glasses since I was eight years old, and my husband was the one who held my eyes open to put them in. If I said I wanted something, he got it for me. That was just the way he was, but now the man who did so much for me is avoiding me. This is the man who went to the doctors with me and heard the same thing I did from them. He turned on me when I needed him the most, because the Superwoman he married was no longer there to carry out our dreams and do the things we had done together.

I know no marriage is perfect, but this is the way I saw ours: We played together, had romantic weekends and shared with each other, created things together, played golf, enjoyed each other. He never argued with me, just said okay and left it alone. One day, however, we reached the place where I had packed my bags to leave because the love of my life started to avoid me by playing golf as much as he could. He started staying out until bedtime. We either argue or just refrain from speaking to one another.

The strain put on our finances by the cost of medication and doctor visits has caused us to seek help. Our savings have diminished. Our lives have turned chaotic, which is stressful. It has gotten to the point where now we are both in therapy because I know he didn't want to live like this, with a wife who can barely get out of bed in the morning, a wife who can't cook anymore or have an intimate relationship with her husband. This illness has caused nothing but stress, anger, helplessness, and pain.

My two sons have dealt with this much better than their dad. The four of us decided to try to get together once a week to keep up-to-date on what is going on in everybody's life. One night I asked them if they could pronounce the name of the disease. The boys said it at the same time, whereas Greg, my husband, couldn't even pronounce the word fibromyalgia. Man, did that hurt me. I've had this condition for four years now, and he still can't pronounce the word. I knew then that he was not on the same page I was on. But now he has started to do things around the house; since we have no money, he can't play golf and hide from me.

▲▲▲

FAMILY

How can we help our family members gain the understanding of our condition that we want them to have? In fact, several good ways exist to educate your loved ones about FM. If you have a husband or partner, invite him or her to meet with your doctor or health-care practitioner. Have the doctor explain FM inside out. Take a list of questions with you that you have gone over with your partner. Check off each item when it has been answered by the doctor. Make sure your partner also asks questions and feels comfortable with the answers.

Read books on FM together (see Resources). There are books on exercise and FM, on diet and FM, on how FM is diagnosed, and on medications and alternative therapies. The Internet is another great resource for information. There is no excuse not to be well-read on this illness.

Consider going to counseling together. Hearing another perspective may help your spouse better understand FM and may help the two of you come to terms with the inevitable changes in your lives wrought by chronic illness.

If you have very young children, it's a good idea to be frank about your condition, but use simple language that they can understand. Perhaps show them a picture illustrating the tender-point sites, and say, "When I have pain, this is where it hurts." Consider using a code phrase that's easier to pronounce than the word *fibromyalgia*. One friend's little boy says he's "feeling puny" when he doesn't feel well. Maybe you could say, "Mommy's feeling puny right now and needs to lie down for a while." Help your kids understand how they can help you—maybe it's by giving you some quiet time when you request it, or maybe it's by playing with a younger sibling while you rest.

Kids worry about whether they will catch your illness, and once they reach a certain age they may also worry about whether you'll die. Tell them the good news about FM—that it is not contagious or fatal, and that you and your doctors are working hard to manage the symptoms so that you'll be able to do some of the fun things you enjoy doing together as a family.

Older children and teenagers may resent the limits your illness imposes on your availability to them. If that seems to be a sticking point, consider arranging a meeting with a family doctor or other adult whom your child trusts, so that he or she can learn more about FM from an outside expert. You might even consider getting counseling with a family therapist. First be sure that the counselor or doctor understands FM. And remember to approach the meeting with a willingness to hear what your kid has to say; it's important that she or he feel heard, too.

If your kids are grown, they may worry about you excessively or feel bad that they can't make you better. A friend whose mother has a serious chronic illness says that her mom periodically reminds her, "Don't bleed for the patient. Don't take on too much of my illness. You have to let me be where I am in my sickness and in my healing process."

Remember, a chronic illness affects everyone in the family. Your role may change as you make room for another presence in your life: that of your illness. Also remember that no matter how well you explain FM, some family members still may have difficulty accepting your limits.

Gerry L. A couple of years ago I changed the status quo. I gave myself permission to say no. I rocked the boat. There was fallout. I knew there would be, but I needed to do this and I needed the full support of my immediate family. I was not going to go down with the ship. Needless to say, there was distress on the part of some family members who were invested in trying to figure out how I could still do things the same way I always had. It really hurts when you hear, "Are you okay? Please stay well, we need you. Please take care of yourself." What that really means is "I want you to do what you have always done for me." It is difficult for my aging family members to understand that our family is growing and adding new members, and that the key is to be flexible. There are always options. We got through it.

At this point I do what is best for me, and then I distance myself. I have a very hard time setting boundaries, but when I forget to do so, I get angry at myself. When that happens, I try to learn from the situation and remember it for the next time.

Marcia D. I notice that by evening my nerves are a little frayed. At times I just need to take time out for myself. I go to my computer or just spend five to ten minutes by myself in the bathroom. I know how bad I feel and a lot of times it's not fair to everybody else. Sometimes I have to stop and look back at my behavior and say, "You're really being a bitch, and it's not fair to the rest of the family, so take five and back off."

If I could change the past, I would do things differently. I have always been independent and have done things for myself and am very impatient. When I want something done, I want it done now, and my family is not geared to that. However, now when I insist on doing everything, usually I pay for it big time. My husband, Joe, is getting better about helping. I think maybe in the last few years he has come to realize that I can't do the things I used to do. His role for years was to come home from work, sit down in his chair, and have his plate put in front of him, and that doesn't happen now.

Sisu G. My role in the family has changed. I'm not sure how. There was a phase when some of my extended family went into denial. "How can she really be sick? Just look at her!" They understand more now, but they are a little leery of me, as if at any moment I might morph into a monster of some kind—some horrible, diseased creature. My family has faced heart disease, cancers, all manner of things. But this illness seems to make people want to pull back, to avoid knowing too much because it's complicated and variable. In my close family, though, my condition seems to have established some level of respect, because they do understand what's happening, and, well, they're proud of me. They know I'm doing a lot in spite of the pain. Especially my mother.

My mother has been the most wonderful help. I keep her posted regularly, and she says I can cry and whine at her whenever I need to about the pain. Which is good—without that outlet, I might go crazy. She is understanding and wise, and this has brought us much closer. Things can get overwhelming, fast, and it's a huge advantage to have her right there, a telephone call away, with advice and the ability to listen patiently. I think FM puts a huge strain on relationships, but healthy ones get stronger and unhealthy ones or weak ones fall apart. Sometimes it's nobody's fault; it just happens.

My extended family has always been a little distant. The hardest part is when people want to play "top this." I'm not interested. They ask me how I am and what's happening to me. After the first half sentence, they break in with an explanation of the latest medical procedure they've undergone. My mum and I call this "the organ recital." And I confess to having occasionally given in to FM—with a hand to my forehead in true swooning style—just to get the hell out of there.

Donna F. My role as a member of my family has not changed—that of mother, maid, cook, nurse, and all the related little things—other than the fact that I need much more help doing the tasks my role requires.

Cydney B. After I quit working, I became the full-time caregiver for my father-in-law, and that was a role I think I cherished, although at the time I didn't know it. It gave me some sense of being needed and having worth. Now it's tough to find that satisfying sense of being needed. No one in the family needs me much anymore, but that comes with age anyway, so it's hard to say how much FM has to do with it.

The children are out of the house now. My younger daughter does not tolerate my limitations well at all. She can't seem to fathom that I am too tired to do something. She recently said that when I first got sick, "We all thought you were just complaining again and were a hypochondriac." I asked her if she thinks that now, and she said no, she knows I am sick. But she still won't cut me any slack.

The older one may have FM. She is terrified of getting it. Her constant complaining about this, that, and the other pain and ache makes me keenly aware of my own complaining (and makes me feel guilty that I may have given her FM).

Victoria M. As recently as last week, my sister-in-law decided that it would be in my best interest to inform me of my "victim mentality": that I doctor-shopped to find things wrong with me and my children in order to seek attention; that I should do something more useful than researching this illness; and that it was about time somebody told me. I had made an effort to rest, dress nicely, and put on makeup to attend a family function, an engagement party. The unsolicited tirade was very distressing. I have put importance on attending my husband's family occasions over the years, for him and for my children, and therefore, because I look okay, it would seem that I must be making all this up! Damned if you do, damned if you don't.

Rachel B. My extended family is in another country. They know I have FM, but they have not seen me yet. I do not know what their reaction will be, and I truly do not know if I want them to see me in this deteriorated state. I know it is hard on them, especially with the diagnosis of MS still not ruled out. My father also has MS and would feel guilty if his daughter was diagnosed with the disease.

Mea C. My mother is just positive that my illness is caused by a food allergy or another type of allergy. All I need to do is get an extensive blood workup so they can find what's causing my FM, and I'll get better.

Penny G. My oldest two children are in their twenties and are not very supportive. They just assume I am okay. My daughter is eleven and we get along well. I still am healthy enough to do things

with her. The things I can't do, my husband does. I think things will
get harder as she gets a few years older.

▲▲▲

REACHING ACCEPTANCE

I can now say I have the full support of my partner, family, and
friends. It wasn't always that way. It took having quite a few long
talks, reading many books, watching educational videos, and continuing with my ongoing research to foster understanding within
the circles of my loved ones. However, it proved well worth it to do
whatever was necessary to explain FM to those close to me. It
helps to realize that before you can introduce FM to your loved
ones, you have to first get past whatever is holding *you* back in
understanding and connecting with your condition.

Acceptance on the part of family members can mean many
things. One state of affairs you probably want to avoid, however, is
an attitude from your loved ones that you're "helpless and hopeless." People's pity—when it translates into attempts to run your
life for you—is not the same thing as their acceptance, compassion, or understanding. I was evaluated by a psychiatrist to see if I
qualified for a particular treatment program. My partner was
closely questioned to see if she "enabled" my illness by doing
things for me so that I could stay in my "chronic-pain behavior."
My partner and I had a good laugh afterwards. She is an R.N. at an
intensive-care burn unit, and unless you are burned or bleeding,
she doesn't have one bit of sympathy. That's just the way I like it.

I always hope that the folks who care about me understand
FM, and if they find they just can't or won't, that's okay, too.

Diane H. I was surprised that after a while my husband not only
believed me but helped me explain to others what having FM was
like. I had two sisters with FM, so the support of my extended family was already there.

Kay B. I rely on my husband, Tim. After two unsuccessful marriages, I have the blessing of a wonderful man. He, too, is afflicted

with illness—hypothyroidism and gout. We often joke that we don't have a complete working body between the two of us! I think my role as a wife is impacted, but Tim is very caring and loving.

Mary H.-B. My relationship with my husband is more fulfilling now than before. He has come to understand that I have limitations and doesn't get upset when I say no. We spend a lot of time talking about the issues that caused me to develop FM/CFS, and he helps me to overcome the issues. He is very supportive of my meditation time and tells me to keep up the work I do for others, since he knows how important that is to me.

Cydney B. My husband and I do less physical stuff together. We have less sex. He gets frustrated with my limitations when he needs help with something that requires my physical participation. On the other hand, he helps me more than he might otherwise, and he accepts me as I am.

Gerry L. My daughter has a very keen sense and can feel how I am doing. She has a real understanding and knows quite a bit about FM. My son and daughter-in-law have great concern and are sensitive to my needs. My children will caution me to not overdo. I know they are both having a hard time dealing with this, each in their own way. I can feel that at times my son doesn't know what to say. But he understands. Mom is always Mom, and I draw deeply for strength to do what I need and want to do for them. That is one of the choices I make. My husband has been there for the roughest times, even though I know he is frustrated and angry that this happened to me and to us.

There have been a few times when I have been alone and have called my daughter or daughter-in-law, shaken, in a lot of pain and fatigue, feeling helpless and afraid. I needed to have that emotional human touch, that connection. Sometimes I could barely speak and would struggle to just say, "Talk to me," until the meds kicked in and some of the fear subsided. It helped. I felt concerned about how my illness was affecting them. They were always reassuring and gentle and did their best to help.

Sondra H. It was hard for my husband to see me suffer and to feel like there was nothing he could instantly do to fix it. My children were scared and unsure. My friends were very understanding. I helped the situation by doing everything I could to learn about the condition and passing what I learned on to others in my life. Information was my best weapon, and it also proved helpful to the doctors treating me that I was an informed patient.

I shared information with my husband, which helped when I didn't do what I should to take care of myself. He'd get me back on track. Sharing information with my kids has brought them so much understanding and has eased their fear. For my friends, I typed a letter. I explained my diagnosis, why I may act or feel a certain way, and why I might not be able to do all the things I used to do. I emphasized that it had nothing to do with how much I valued our relationship. This was very important, because for some time we were unable to get together with friends due to my health. I didn't want to lose those relationships while I worked through the changes I had to make in my life.

FRIENDS

Take time to educate your friends about FM. Sometimes friends are hesitant to ask questions that need to be addressed. Tell your friends right up front, "This is what fibromyalgia is all about," or simply sit down with them one-on-one and invite them to ask questions. I have found that people are open to listening about FM if the information is presented in a way that's easy to understand. Show them several books and take your time. It's never too late to take this step.

Recently, my brother asked me if I was having a hard day. It means a lot to me that he understands what makes a good or bad day, and I was grateful that he had taken the time to find out about fibromyalgia. Even if you have had a bad experience explaining the illness to people, the rewards are great when you finally make a connection with someone about the issue, so keep trying.

Alison H. I think some people still feel that I'm faking everything. But those closely involved in my everyday life have a good grasp on what is going on, and they accept the fact that I cannot do all the things I used to do. There are times when I myself don't accept it, but then my friends help me realize that things happen for a reason.

Losing Friendships to FM

Even while you work hard to educate your friends about FM, and even while you hope in your heart that each of them will reach acceptance about your condition, it's important to realize that some of your friendships may fail to survive this major life change.

Katie G. The old saying that you really know who your friends are in a crisis is very true. I have fewer friends than before, but they're all high quality. How many relationships can we really nurture and attend to with any intimacy, anyway? Some people fled me when I got sick, almost as though they could get it. Some were disgusted and frustrated and basically told me to snap out of it. Others who were high achievers and movers and shakers had no way to relate to me, as I wasn't "on their level" any more. I felt with some friends and family members that I was an embarrassment to them. Here I had so much education and had achieved a lot yet was saying that I couldn't get out of bed and felt like I had the flu all the time. I couldn't go out or attend events; I had to cancel at the last minute. People told me I was unreliable.

On the other hand, I have become a very good friend to myself. That has been an important result of this illness. I have time (often because I do not move a muscle) to reflect and, while being quiet, to really think things through.

Sisu G. My friends have had to adjust to the same things I have: my lack of energy, my pain, my inability to keep up. My circle of friends fell apart fast when I got sick. Most of them were people my own age, with whom I liked to do things. Now that I can't hang out at a club, go hiking, or stay up all night talking, they simply don't have as much impetus to hang out with me. I'm a project; I'm a chore. It's true that the ones who left were only social-level friends, but everyone needs a few of those, just to help them feel normal.

Some of the friends I lost were people I genuinely cared about who couldn't face watching me go through this. They'd known me for years and had watched me always be the strongest person they knew. And then suddenly—I wasn't. (I am still strong, but it's different; it's all internal now.) They went away. They didn't just vanish; they drifted, mostly. Stopped calling, stopped answering calls. Some of them I miss very much. I have other friends now; I have met some splendid people who understand. But I miss having my health not be an issue.

My remaining friends are true and dear, and I have learned to be a great deal more patient with them. I found out early on that the best way to deal with things was to keep everyone posted. I'd send out bulletins on what was happening with me. Every one of my friends knows what FM is and how it gets treated, which spares a lot of wasted time. I tell them it's like having very bad arthritis, and they understand that concept pretty well. I send updates by e-mail when I go to the doctors, and my friends are just wonderful in response. They give me very little pity, yet a lot of understanding. So I don't have anyone to give me a back rub, but I do have someone to whom I can talk about doctors and medicines and tests, without worrying about instilling panic. And it means that when I am able to go out and do things, I can do so and feel like a normal person. That's worth a lot to me.

I know that this illness destroys a lot of relationships, and I know that I certainly don't have the energy to pursue a normal dating life. I wish I did. There are still a lot of people who make advances and who aren't frightened off by my illness. But I'm just not up to it, and even if I were, I'm still stuck on this one person, so I guess I'm managing to have a typical life after all.

Nancy D.   There are many examples of how I pruned my friend-ship tree. I am no longer scared of losing a friend. It is no longer an unthinkable thought. I recognize that I have gained many of the wonderful things about that person, and I know they will miss me more than they think they will. I have also found that I love being alone. That is a good start.

When to Tell?

One of the things FM'ers must consider is when—if ever—is the right time to disclose their chronic condition to people outside their immediate circle of family and friends.

Nancy D. I have learned to be more aware of whom I tell about my illness. Every person does not have to know and see every side of me. I am multidimensional and evolving into a person I like a lot better. I have made changes that not every friend has liked.

Rachel B. My friends know me and know I have FM. My new friends got introduced to the symptoms during my last flare-up, yet I am always very resistant to their seeing me in this state. I have great support from my friends, but I feel that I put an extra burden upon them. I do not want to be a burden to my friends. I love them too dearly for that, and I do not want to jeopardize my friendships due to the strain the disease can put on a relationship.

Sondra H. There are so many people whom I work with or deal with who have no idea of my condition, and to me that's an accomplishment. I don't want to be labeled by FM; there's much more to me than that.

DATING

To date or not? It depends on your energy level and your own acceptance of the illness. I have heard women say that dating just wasn't worth the initial energy expenditure and the effort required to sustain another friendship in the long haul. When I hear this argument, I always say, "Why not run a personal ad?" That way, you can tell the other person before you meet him or her what your requirements and needs are. You can work out some of the details ahead of time.

Example: "Single, mature, thirty-five-year-old woman, homebody, loves the slow-paced life. Available during the day; open for movies with a calm, kind individual, etc." Or you might even consider being candid in the ad about having a chronic illness. If you do, anyone who responds to the ad is at least somewhat prepared to deal with potential lifestyle restrictions. You could add a sentence like the following to your ad: "Learning to live positively and constructively with a chronic health condition." Of course, making such a choice goes back to the question of how much about your FM to divulge to whom, and when. Such decisions are different for everyone; only you know the best way for you to proceed.

I think personal ads are terrific, especially the ones that require your potential date to write to you in order to introduce himself. That way, you can tell immediately if he has a brain and good communication skills. Second, you can chat over the phone to see if there is a connection. Third, arrange a face-to-face date—in a public place, for safety.

However you phrase your ad, when prospective dates call, be up-front. Tell them you have a chronic-pain illness and require rest at times. Disclose what you are comfortable with, and then go out and have some fun. FM doesn't rule your life, and it certainly needn't isolate you as a single person if that is not what you want. If you are lonely, you don't have to be alone.

Cybill C. I date now, and my dates are informed early in the game about FM. I have had FM for so long that my kids have adapted. They know that sometimes I am too sick to do things. Luckily, I have a very supportive family. My friends are great, too.

Katie G. After I was forced to stop working, my boyfriend and I broke up. He said the illness was part of it. The frustrating part of dating is determining when and how much you reveal. To some men, I have been very straightforward and matter-of-fact. Some are frightened by it; fewer are not. When I did hold back and just said I was taking time off from work, the needling I got was enough to make me say, "Don't call me anymore." They acted like I was lazy or the queen. Little did they know. Even if I don't say anything, it seems to intrigue them all the more. I walk a fine line. I like being honest and up-front, but it doesn't always work, especially now that I haven't been employed since March of 1995.

Sisu G.   About my love life? I can't go on many dates because I haven't the energy. One guy whom I've been trying to stay in contact with for two years in the longest game of telephone tag thought I was making it all up as an excuse not to date him. I have to explain every time. I have gone out on a few dates, but it's more of an effort than it otherwise would be.

▲▲▲

A SUPPORT NETWORK

No matter how your loved ones react to your diagnosis, you need a support network—that is, a person or persons you can phone when you're feeling blue about your health, or when you need some practical feedback, such as discussing the pros and cons of a new line of treatment. I find it especially helpful to stay involved with a circle of friends who have FM; they know exactly what I'm talking about because they've been there too. If you are lucky enough to have a support group in your hometown, I highly recommend attending at least one meeting to see if it offers the right kind of support for you. (Read about support groups in Chapter 3.)

Some women, however, draw their support from a network of family, friends, and neighbors.

Nancy D.   My support network is now fine-tuned. It is the link that makes me feel important to others, because they continually show their thanks for having me around. The key people in my network are my son, my parents, relatives, friends (the best of the crop), a wonderful FM/CFS support-group leader who has become a friend and is continually inspirational, doctors, e-mail friends, neighborly neighbors, and my polite community.

Jean T.   Another group of my supporters includes my friends where I live. Several of us like to go to lunch somewhere nice a couple of times a month. Since I can't put my walker in my trunk, I have to let them do it for me. They are also good enough to check in with each other every day to be sure everyone is okay.

The couple who are the managers of the building where I live are also a part of my support network. Even though it isn't in their job description, they are so considerate and helpful. I rely on them a lot. It gives me a feeling of security just to know they are there.

Gerry L.   My support network is kind of split into two different worlds. I've stepped into a world of care providers who believe in homeopathic, complementary medicine. So I have family and friends, and then those in this other world who have become family and friends.

In addition, I have a very dear friend who has cancer, and we have been there for each other through all our trials, joys, and life events for some thirty-five years. She even got acupuncture because I nudged her to try it, and it helped her. She is a hero. She has been a tremendous source of strength and comfort right from the beginning. She has moved to Florida. We miss each other. Over the past few years, as we both were suffering in our own ways, we laughed and cried together. She would get angry with me because I didn't call her when I needed to. We have spent many nights talking on the phone at 2:00 or 3:00 A.M. She supported everything I did, right from the start. She was interested and wanted to understand and rejoiced with me when there was some success or I had several good days in a row. She has been a comfort and a loyal friend. I can't fool her.

Rachel B.   Living in a small, rural town does not provide many support-group opportunities. My support network consists of very close friends who provide their assistance to me and my partner. I'm happy that our new friends include my partner by asking her how she is coping or holding up. I know in the past she struggled because all the attention was going to me and nobody considered the fact that her life has also been changed since the onset of my symptoms.

Alison H.   My support network is my family, my friend, and the message board. They all are very helpful and willing to help me understand what is going on. They are as eager as I am to understand how this affects my body. My family and friends have done extensive research and ask a lot of questions. Participating in the message board shows me that there are people out there who are worse off than I am. These same people give me great coping techniques. They also just listen, and sometimes I need that from someone who truly knows that I'm not crazy!

The most important people in my support circle, however, are my mom and my best friend. They take the time to try and figure all this stuff out.

Charlene M. I have a very close friend whom I can call any time, day or night. My family knows what is wrong, but they can't understand why one minute I seem fine and the next I have to lie down. So I need to have someone who understands that I require time to get past my flare.

▲▲▲

Dealing with the people you're closest to can be one of the greatest challenges of living with fibromyalgia. But the sense of connection fostered when you and a loved one reach a place of mutual acceptance and understanding about your illness can also yield great rewards. For that reason, don't give up on educating your family and friends about FM. Once they're firmly in your corner, they can be your strongest support.

Dealing with Doctors and Other Health-Care Providers

In Chapter 3 we touched on the importance for FM patients of establishing a relationship with a doctor or other primary-care provider who will partner with us in our health care. In this chapter we explore what such a partnership entails, as well as other issues related to dealing with the people we're paying to help us care for ourselves: how to find a good doctor, informing ourselves in preparation for our doctor appointments, financial concerns, and establishing a relationship of mutual trust and confidence with our health-care providers.

As consumers of medical care, we have responsibilities. We educate ourselves before buying a car or a refrigerator; it makes sense that it's even more important to inform ourselves before purchasing care for our bodies and minds. Stated another way, and as expressed repeatedly throughout this book, a patient's true primary-care provider is herself. This chapter aims to help clarify our responsibilities as patients versus those of the medical professionals in whom we place our trust.

FINDING A DOCTOR

Finding a doctor with whom you are comfortable and who has a good understanding of FM is a challenge, yet doing so at the onset of your illness is of utmost importance. Wasting time, money, and precious energy on a doctor who doesn't understand FM or has very little time to spend with you is a pitfall you want to avoid. Once you do find a primary-care doctor you think is the right one for you, establishing a relationship of mutual trust takes time, but it is worth the effort to do so, because she or he will become a very important part of your health-care team.

FM patients don't always end up with a rheumatologist as their primary-care provider. As our correspondents write in this chapter, the medical practitioners who diagnosed them and who treat them come from many different backgrounds. They include general practitioners, neurologists, rheumatologists, chiropractors, even a podiatrist. It doesn't matter how you found your doctor or what type of doctor he or she is as long as you feel you are making progress and being treated well. If that is the case, you have made a good choice.

There are several ways to begin your search for a doctor who specializes in treating FM, including:

◀ Getting suggestions from support-group members or other FM friends;

◀ Physician referral. An ethical doctor will tell you up front if he or she feels that he or she is not the best-qualified professional to treat your condition. In such cases the doctor often can recommend another physician by name;

◀ The local phone book. Some doctors specializing in hard-to-treat conditions such as FM carry large ads in the yellow pages listing their specialties;

◀ Fibromyalgia (or related) organizations and websites. The American College of Rheumatology website (www.rheumatology.org) includes a directory of rheumatologists

by location. The Fibromyalgia Network (website www.
fmnetnews.com; [800] 853-2929) offers a physician-
referral service;

◀ Your insurance plan. Consult the directory of your plan's
preferred providers. Such lists are often organized by the
doctors' specialties. You might start your search under the
heading "rheumatology";

◀ "Ask-a-nurse" hotline. Some hospitals or medical centers
sponsor these toll-free phone numbers so that anyone in
the community can get basic medical questions answered
by an R.N. They may be able to provide you with a list of
rheumatologists, chiropractors, or other FM specialists in
your region.

To help you determine whether a particular doctor is experienced in treating FM and is a good match for you, call and ask her
or him a few basic questions before you even schedule an appointment. You might start with the following:

◀ What is your usual protocol for treating FM?

◀ Do you have other FM patients, and are they making
progress?

◀ Will you listen to my suggestions and be a partner in my
health care?

You will be able to tell quickly if a doctor doesn't believe in
FM or doesn't know enough about it to do you any good. Watch
out for doctors who focus only on your mental health or nurses
and office managers who don't follow up with your test results or
who treat you as if you are a complainer. Remember, *you* are the
boss in this situation. Your doctor is providing a service that *you*
pay for.

Mary H.-B. I was diagnosed in September 1998 by a chiropractor
I found in the yellow pages. I woke up one morning and couldn't
get out of bed because I was in so much pain due to stress at the

office; I had to be lifted out of bed just to go to the bathroom. That's what made me decide to look for a chiropractor.

Donna F. I was diagnosed in 1997 by a doctor I found online. I decided to go to a doctor because I could not understand or live with the sudden relentless, merciless, tortuous pain and burning sensation I was experiencing. It felt as though I had aged thirty years overnight. The doctor who diagnosed me has a good, respectable reputation, and I support that.

BE INFORMED: PREPARING FOR YOUR DOCTOR APPOINTMENT

As soon as you have secured an appointment with a doctor, begin to take notes. Write down the following:

◀ When did you begin to feel ill? Some folks know the exact date when their "flulike symptoms" began (and their old life ended). For others, it's the date of the accident or trauma that seemed to lead to FM

◀ Did the symptoms come on suddenly or over time?

◀ Any dates of hospitalization for any reason

◀ Any medications you are currently taking, including dosages and side effects

◀ Any supplements you are currently taking, including dosages and side effects

◀ Sleep patterns and difficulties

◀ Description of your pain levels

If you must wait a few weeks to see the doctor, make the most of the time by charting your sleep, pain, and exercise habits. Begin your list as soon as you know the appointment date so you can write down ideas and questions as they come up, and add to the list as your appointment draws closer. This allows you time to notice changes in your body so you can apprise the doctor easily.

Being prepared for your appointment takes away some of the stress of meeting a doctor for the first time. Having a list or notes will indicate that you are a patient who is knowledgeable and serious about getting the best care possible. Being prepared also assures you of not wasting any time in getting right down to what treatments to try for your illness.

If you feel your doctor doesn't take enough time for you, it's very important to let him or her know that. Each patient requires a different level of support and care. It's up to you to voice your concerns; do this by writing a letter or calling and requesting a few moments on the phone with your doctor. If your doctor isn't open to this, it's a clue to how he or she will treat you in the future.

In the beginning of my illness, I had numerous questions for my rheumatologist, a big list each time I went in. Now I see him every other month for pain management and medication follow-up. Still, I always make sure to have a list of questions and observations when seeing him. He is a very busy doctor who specializes in FM, and his office is always full and bustling. But my time with him is very important to me, and I am assured of his attention when I am checking off each question and suggestion. It's an awful feeling to leave the doctor's office feeling you don't understand why you are being asked to try a new drug or that you didn't have enough time to explain something new that is happening to you.

Patients who have undergone several ineffective treatments or therapies can seem demanding in their search for relief. Unrelieved pain can cause depression and fear. I have been a patient like this. One medication after another either didn't work or caused side effects that were impossible to live with. I felt out of control, and my doctor at the time questioned whether it was depression or FM that was causing so much anguish.

Currently, I don't require the support I once did. I use the Internet and an occasional support-group meeting if I want to know about new treatments. If they sound promising, I ask my doctor about them. Many times he has cautioned me to wait until the research substantiates the hype for a new treatment; other times, if he knows the treatment is sound and scientifically researched, he will determine if it is appropriate for me to try.

Sondra H. It is so very, very important to be an informed patient. Your health-care professionals appreciate it so much. You only get a small window of their time, and, generally, people fail to ask the right questions and to provide the answers the doctors are seeking. A good relationship and partnership with your health-care providers is crucial.

Val T. I believe we all need to be our own best advocates in our health care and to research the treatment plans and medications our providers prescribe. The more we know, the better off we will be! We know our bodies far better than anyone else.

Sisu G. Here are a few pointers for getting the most out of your relationship with your medical providers:

◢ Don't think of doctors as mechanics. Think of them as plant specialists. Your body does not get fixed like a car; it grows like a plant. You bring it to the doctors to find out what's wrong and to get a plan for how to deal with the problem, and then you treat it in lots of small ways that change the overall balance of health.

◢ Figure out what your biggest issues are before you go to the doctor.

◢ Get a full copy of your medical record. This is essential so you'll have it if you ever need to see a different doctor.

My rheumatologist is very good. He's made it clear that if I ever have an issue, I am to call him, and I do. He really meant it when he took his Hippocratic oath. He is a very busy man. I see him every three months, although his office will make time if something new is happening to me. Once he called on a Sunday night in response to a call I'd made about my medication, even though he was on a lecture tour at the time. He says that a lot of patients never come back once they have the diagnosis, or they come back with an attitude of, "That didn't work; fix me properly this time." This is very frustrating for him, I would imagine. I have a lot of respect for him. He treats me more like a student than like a person to be repaired.

I go in with my notes and my status report, and we talk about what's happening to me. We talk about what can be done, and he always is careful to leave the final decision regarding treatment options up to me. He asks what we should focus on. Right now, it's pain management. It used to be sleep. We talk about what to try, and I follow his recommendation. I call him if things aren't working, and we go through the same process again. Studying, reading, and taking a real interest in how things are happening inside me have benefited me at the doctor's office. With my doctor, I've been able to tailor a treatment program that helps me. I feel as if I am in control of my illness, which makes a big difference.

Charlene M. I have learned that I can be very insistent when I am in pain and need some help. I also have learned that I need other people to help me, and now I am willing to ask them.

Jean T. I print out pertinent information I find on the Internet and take it to my doctor, along with a list of any questions I have. He always takes me seriously and does anything he can to try to help the pain. He has a big hug for me whenever I am ready to go home. I appreciate his caring.

Donnie M. I grew up believing that doctors were little gods, and boy have I changed my opinion about that. I now feel that in order to survive, we more or less have to do the best we can at being our own doctor. By this I mean we have to try and put the pieces together and to figure out what medications work best for us, and we certainly are the ones who have to remember our own medical history. After all, we are only allowed our fifteen minutes, which is not enough time for the doctor to review our full history. I carry a written list when I go in for my appointments so I do not forget anything I need to discuss, and to discourage the doctor from rushing me out the door until I have finished going down my list.

FINANCIAL CONCERNS: IS IT WORTH PAYING OUT-OF-POCKET?

When my rheumatologist left my HMO plan, I followed him. I am now a self-pay patient. Yes, it is expensive, but I know I am getting excellent care from the doctor who knows me best. Acupuncture and chiropractic care are sometimes covered by insurance, but most people pay out-of-pocket for these treatments. In my opinion, such specialists are just as important as your primary-care doctor, and they function just as much as part of your health-care team.

Most FM patients have a team that may include:

◄ Primary-care doctor or rheumatologist

◄ Acupuncturist or chiropractor

◄ Body worker, myotherapist, Feldenkrais or Alexander Technique practitioner, or massage therapist

◄ Exercise physiotherapist

◄ Mental-health counselor

These treatments can be expensive, and not every treatment will work for every FM patient. Still, as you can afford to, consider trying something new. Many treatments can be done at home once you learn how, such as physical-therapy exercises, yoga, and movement therapies. This is a time to trust your instincts. If you have a limited budget, don't try an expensive new therapy that you're uncomfortable with. Talk over complementary treatments with your doctor and support group. Many yoga and exercise practitioners offer free classes you can attend on a trial basis. That way, you can experiment without breaking the bank. (See Chapter 5 for more discussion of complementary treatments for FM.)

Rae H. If we had better medical coverage or a better income, I would establish a relationship with an energy worker, a naturopath, and a massage therapist, as I believe they would provide the most holistic intervention.

Emma L. I am mad that my HMO doctor was not more interested in helping me. I regret that I was never financially able to consistently seek other doctors' help. I regret that I did not pursue being treated by other doctors in spite of being unable to afford it at the time. I felt too responsible and reasonable over ten years of health disaster to risk financial disaster as well.

EXPECTATIONS IN CARE

You have a right to expect good health care. If you belong to an HMO, it's true that there are rules to follow, but, generally, if you and the doctor you are assigned to aren't a good match, you can usually try someone else within the system.

I am always surprised to learn of women who blindly go to an unknown doctor and then remain as a patient with that doctor even if they fail to get good results. If you find that your doctor doesn't listen, doesn't take suggestions, or is condescending, do not waste any more time. Pay your bill, get your records, and look for another doctor.

Included in this section are stories of patients who have had "bad doctor" experiences. It seems as if most chronic-pain patients have at least one story about a doctor who treated them with disrespect or who didn't believe in FM. It's instructive to realize that doctors are just like anyone else. They want to successfully treat their patients and return them to good health. When FM patients describe their pain, doctors have to interpret the pain. How do they do this? By imposing their own ideas of what pain is. Treating FM is complicated by the fact that most doctors tend to see people who are in acute pain rather than chronic pain. In addition, they may hold beliefs and biases, as well as a fear of the patient's possible addiction to pain medications.

Kay B. I was sent to a rheumatologist who handed me a pamphlet on FM, and the light went on over my head. I tested positive for eighteen out of eighteen tender points. He treated me for a

short time, and when I showed no improvement he told me I didn't
want to get any better. So our professional relationship was severed. He was fired approximately one year after this, because his
patients complained to the clinic board of standards and practices
about his lack of empathy.

Gerry L. I trust my doctors and their judgment, but getting there
is a process. I trust their knowledge, dedication, and research, and
I trust my gut. I've been to enough doctors that it doesn't take long
to figure out who to stop seeing. If they don't like being questioned
or have too much ego, then they're not the one for me. I saw an
ear, nose, and throat specialist who told me it was just quackery,
that any doctor who told me he or she could help was just telling
me what I wanted to hear. He told me to go home and live with it. I
never went to him again.

Rae H. I was very fortunate to connect with a physician in the
clinic where I received my medical care. Unfortunately, he moved
out of state. I called another rheumatologist, but his staff advised
me that "there is nothing that can be done about FM, and he really
doesn't want to deal with it." This was quite an eye-opener regarding the variability of how practitioners might respond to FM.

Wendy K. I currently see a primary-care physician. I started to
see him after I fired my previous doctor, who I'm sure doesn't
believe in FM. The previous doctor, after I told her that Ultram
didn't help my pain at all, told me that she had "no more tricks up
her sleeve." She would not prescribe pain meds.

Victoria M. I do not trust medicos in general. I have found so
many irregularities in test results which have gone unnoticed or
ignored. I have diplomatically questioned this on occasion and
been bewildered by the holier-than-thou attitude of these specialists and caregivers. I have been shocked by the brazen and defiant
way in which so-called health professionals cruelly and piously
judge individuals. I tell them, "I am sick, not stupid."

Nancy D. I saw a new primary-care physician, who changed my
hormone medication but flat out refused to continue to refill Zoloft,
and cut me off cold turkey from cyclobenzaprine (Flexeril). I have

been on cyclobenzaprine for years. If I hadn't had an emergency "stash" built up, I would have been in really bad pain with leg cramps, or I might have had to go to the emergency room. After I spoke to his nurse about this, he did not return my call. I had supplied this doctor with medical records, a list of symptoms, and a list of medications during my first visit.

Cybill C. I have had a rheumatologist who didn't seem to take me or my symptoms seriously, so I chose not to return to him.

Donnie M. In 1995 or 1996, I was taken to the ER twice for rapid heartbeat. I had severe fatigue. If I tried to move from my bed, my heart rate would go up. I had absolutely no energy, could not drive, and sometimes could not even shower, brush my teeth, or walk. The headaches were so intense, I felt suicidal. My husband had to take off work, drive forty-five minutes home, and take me to my doctor. I had to lean on my husband to walk into the doctor's office. We did this several times, only to hear that there was nothing wrong with me.

I cannot tell you how many times I was told it was all in my head, or that I was "at that age," or asked if there was any stress in my life, etc. When I kept insisting that the doctor continue to do tests, he finally ordered one more blood test. This one showed a high sedimentation rate—which measures blood coagulation to detect infections, inflammatory diseases, tissue destruction, and other conditions—and on that basis he misdiagnosed me with polymyalgia rheumatica.

After the diagnosis of polymyalgia rheumatica, I was put on prednisone and told if I did not take it I might go blind, and there would be nothing the doctors could do. After about a year and a half of taking prednisone, I was in a pitiful state. My body and face were swollen, and I had bruises on my arms and legs. I felt as bad as ever or maybe even worse. When the specialist wanted to again increase the prednisone, I refused and went to UCLA to see a new specialist, the best thing I have ever done for myself. The new doctor did a thorough physical, including blood tests, and then diagnosed me with FM, saying I never had polymyalgia rheumatica.

It is important for us to discern the difference between a doctor who is trying hard to help us and is frustrated because there seems to be little change in our condition, and a doctor who is frustrated to be dealing with us, period. FM patients often need help in finding alternative treatments for pain, adjustments in dosages of medications when side effects become too much to bear, and support when the pain is out of control. A doctor's level of skill in handling these subtle issues highlights the difference between one who is adept at dealing with patients suffering chronic pain and one who is better at treating acute pain.

One of the best doctors on my health-care team is my chiropractor, Robert J. Freitas, D.C. He is open to anything new that is medically sound, always takes the time to listen, and stays current on the newest treatments by going to seminars. Here, he tells of his own frustrations about making a difference in the lives of his fibromyalgia patients:

> I have been practicing as a chiropractor for twenty years. In that time I have been accustomed to seeing injured patients and either being able to improve their condition or referring them elsewhere for further workup and appropriate care.
>
> It has been my experience that patients with FM don't always get better. The treatment I give them appears to provide symptomatic relief for very short periods of time. I have become more and more frustrated that I cannot find a treatment protocol that offers these individuals a less painful way of life.
>
> As physicians, we are taught to find the problem and fix it. With FM patients, that principle goes out the window. I have to accept that any small amount of relief I can give them helps. It would be easy to tell them that what I have to offer is not curative and to send them on their way. But according to patient feedback, a little relief is helpful, even if it's only temporary.
>
> I would say to any chiropractor who is treating people with FM, "Don't get discouraged." Continue to give them what you can, study new techniques, both nutritional and physical, and read about what others are doing.

Dr. Freitas's final comments can apply to FM patients, too: Even if your expectations of effective treatment leave you frustrated with the care you're receiving, don't get discouraged. Continue through trial and error to look for the right health-care practitioners, keep studying and learning about new ways to help yourself, and stay plugged in to what other FM'ers and their doctors are doing.

ESTABLISHING TRUST

Kathleen J. Armitage, M.D., F.R.C.P., is a specialist in physical medicine and rehabilitation (physiatrist), with a practice in Ontario, Canada. She is author of *The ABC Workbook of Fibromanagement for Fibromyalgia* (see Resources). Here she shares her thoughts on patients' confidence in their health providers:

> Confidence is key to developing trust, and by that I mean both confidence in yourself and confidence in your caregiver. Finding confidence in your caregiver is a challenge in our society. We are challenged constantly to be cautious about whom we get our care from. We are challenged constantly to get a second opinion. We are aware that medical professionals make errors. I think trusting the medical advice we receive is very difficult when we hear contrary opinions.
>
> Trust is a crucial ingredient in a good relationship with a service provider, whether we are trusting that person to fix our car, cut our hair, or provide medical treatment. It is something that must be established between the client and the caregiver, or between the patient and the physician, yet it is also something the patient must develop herself. I don't think there is any way someone can infuse another person with the ability to trust. Somewhere along the line we have to trust that the other person has our interests at heart. Confidence is the centerpiece of the management plan for fibromyalgia.

Trusting a doctor takes time. First we want to see if the doctor will treat us with respect and listen to our ideas. Doctors earn a patient's trust by being available, interested, knowledgeable, and caring.

Rachel B. I trust my primary-care physician. He listens to me and discusses possible next steps. He does not want to put me on a lot of drugs and wants to fight the cause instead of the symptoms. He's as frustrated with the disease as I am and would do everything in his power to find a solution.

Gerry L. I trust my rheumatologist. He does not judge. He is definitely traditional and truly dedicated. He has studied FM for sixteen years. He respects the fact that there are certain meds I will not take. He knows I research everything. He has had to convince me of the difference between addiction and dependence. He also shows an interest in the alternative treatments I have undertaken and that have helped me. He will give me his honest opinion, and I believe he has partnered with me. He understands my pain, fatigue, and other symptoms.

Cheryl R. I trust my doctor completely. He seems to have great concern for my health and to believe my problems. He not only treats me like a person but allows me to have a say in my treatment. He is kind and caring.

YOU AND YOUR PHYSICIAN:
A PARTNERSHIP

We know that FM is a complex syndrome affecting many of the major systems in our body. For this reason, it seems to me that relying on one doctor to care for us may not be the most complete way to go.

I rely on my rheumatologist for medication for pain, sleep, and depression. I rely on my chiropractor for pain relief and to keep my spine in good order. My exercise physiotherapist helps me keep my muscles lengthened and strong so I don't hurt myself. And my mental-health counselor helps me to cope with living with a chronic-pain condition.

However, it's my responsibility to care for myself and to adjust to life with FM. No doctor can teach me what I already know; it's my body and I must decide what medications to put in it and how best to take care of myself. Luckily, I have great support for doing this in my team of health-care practitioners.

Below, the women tell us about their successes in partnering with their health-care providers to live well with FM.

Lalenya R. My rheumatologist is my primary physician for FM. She is a very caring, intelligent, and resourceful person whose only focus is FM. She relays important information from her research, and she never rushes her exam.

Nancy D. My pain-clinic doctor now sees three patients total, and I am certain it is at his expense. I am lucky to be one of those three, because no doctors here are taking new patients. This doctor prescribes methadone and alprazolam (Xanax). He feels confidence in me because I keep learning and I don't have addictive behavior. He spends a lot of time with me and covers every symptom and asks a lot of questions. When I told him I wanted off the fentanyl patches and opioids altogether and wanted to try methadone, he said it made a lot of sense to him. He researched and customized the right conversion for me.

Cybill C. I mostly rely on my primary-care doctor. He is very open to trying new treatments, and he reinforced that FM is not all in my head. Unlike other doctors, he was vigilant about getting to the root of the problems and not just treating the symptoms. We have a very good relationship. He is very honest about the fact that he is not an expert on FM. I frequently give him articles on the subject.

Ginger C. My primary-care physician is my internal-medicine M.D. He made the original diagnosis of FM. I had one referral to a rheumatologist, who agreed with the treatment plan suggested by my M.D. I completely trust my M.D. He is open to information I give him, and he listens to any questions, concerns, or ideas I might have. He has been very understanding, and he makes sure I am getting good pain control. He is very thorough and compassionate.

Jean T.   My doctor is due a lot of credit. He is the most understanding, considerate doctor I have ever had. He has never told me there was no such thing as FM, as so many other doctors have.

Norah T.   My doctor and I have a love/hate relationship that his nurses say is like no other he has. He has prescribed narcotics for ten years against his inclination, sometimes is generous if I need more, sometimes is a bastard about it. We are friends; we share life information as well. It's primarily a good fit.

Charlene M.   My doctor and I have a good relationship. After going to all of the specialists and also talking to him, I decided I would just see him unless something crops up about which we both decide I need to see a specialist. He lets me help make decisions.

Nancy D.   The bottom line is this: The person I rely on most for primary care is me.

Nancy's comment sums up the spirit of proactive self-care: Hold high but realistic expectations of your health-care providers, and at the same time realize that it's up to you to learn how to live well with fibromyalgia.

CHAPTER
10

Dealing with the Rest
of the World

This chapter addresses how to handle expectations from people outside of one's immediate circle of family and friends, including employers and coworkers, and that nebulous "they," society in general. Perhaps most important, it discusses the importance of giving ourselves a break. After all, when we're feeling secure and confident in our own decisions, we worry much less about whether others "approve" of us.

SOCIETAL EXPECTATIONS

There is enormous pressure in our society to be healthy and productive. The 1950s notion of the "ideal family," composed of the father who is the breadwinner and the mother who stays at home taking care of 2.5 kids, has given way to many different sorts of families. A woman today is increasingly likely to live with the stress of being a single, working mom, but even if her family profile consists of two parents and their offspring living under one roof, there is pressure on her to hold down a job outside of the home while maintaining the role of mother, being active in her religion, doing volunteer work, exercising, and making time for friends and family. For women living with a debilitating chronic illness such as fibromyalgia, the expectations to keep all these balls in the air can feel demoralizing.

Rae H. There are definitely societal pressures. I believe it might have been easier to be a woman with FM decades ago, before we climbed on the tightrope of trying to balance careers and family. For women of generations past, working was a choice, not an obligation.

Cybill C. As a woman in this society, a lot of responsibilities are placed on me. Even though we have evolved, it is still traditional for the woman to work, take care of the kids, and do the cooking, cleaning, and laundry. All of those responsibilities are overwhelming to someone with FM, when a good day means just being able to get out of bed. I become ecstatic when I am well enough to vacuum.

Cydney B. There is the pressure to be some sort of contributing member of society. It's crushing to meet new people. What's the first question a new acquaintance asks? "What do you do?" I still can't answer that. "I do nothing," I say. What more is there to say? "Surely you do something," they say. I can't even keep house well! And I still always rankle at being labeled "homemaker" on forms as soon as I say I don't work. I am a lousy homemaker because I am sick. Therefore, what am I? How do I fill out the form? To make myself feel good, I often say I am a writer, but it's been three years since I have had anything published or even submitted anything.

Mary H.-B. I feel a lot of pressure, especially from other women. They treat me as if this were all in my head. Right now I'm thirty five weeks pregnant with my fourth child, and my supervisor at work asked me why I am having children if I have a condition that causes me to require accommodations so I can work from home. My office coworkers are very resentful that I work most of my week from home. They think I'm lying about my illness just so I don't have to come into the office. This is an issue that I'm working on. I'm learning to see people for who they are and how to not let their issues get to me.

Nancy D. The comments people have made to me have been overwhelmingly torturous. A person once invited me to a luncheon, and in front of a table of eight I was introduced with, "This is

Nancy, she's, uh, unemployed." Another comment I have heard several times that hurts a lot is, "Unlike you, I still have to work for a living."

▲▲▲

As touched on earlier in the book, every FM patient I have spoken with has a story to tell about a time when someone denied the validity of their illness by saying, "But you look so good!" or, "How long will it be until you return to work?" I had just been diagnosed with FM and CFS, and I stopped by my workplace to tell my employers and colleagues that *finally* I knew what was wrong with me. A coworker asked me to tell her about the illnesses. As I described them, she looked closely at me and said, "But it can't be too long until you get back to work. After all, I've been fatigued chronically many times in my life, and I was always able to bounce back. Could it just be depression?"

People are used to seeing someone who's sick either get better or die. When an illness goes on and on, they don't readily accept it or understand why. Like all others with an invisible illness characterized by chronic pain, we must find a way to answer these probably well-meaning, but still very distressing, questions.

Ginger C. I have experienced societal pressure in the form of disbelief or questions when I tell someone I can't do something because of my health. At times there is an unspoken attitude of "You don't look sick."

Katie G. Some people have actually said to my face that I look so good, I must be faking it. Faking?! No moron in the world would or could fake this. I refuse to look sick—that is, to let my hair, appearance, or body go to pot. Taking excellent care of oneself and one's body promotes a more positive self-image. Granted, I do not shower or wash my hair every day, and sometimes I go a week without makeup, unheard of prior to my illness.

I've also been told that I was lucky I didn't have cancer or AIDS or that I wasn't in the hospital with machines hooked into me. People have said I was fortunate and should be happy I could walk, move around, and do things. They entirely missed the point. They may have been trying to console me or make me feel better, but their comments only contributed to my aloneness. I've been told "Everyone has problems" or "Just get over it and stop complaining." The Irish-Catholic stiff-upper-lip mentality does nothing for me.

Lalenya R. If I had a dreaded disease that showed up in a blood test or X ray, people would tend to be more supportive.

ADAPTING AT WORK

You may have to continue working for financial reasons, or you may want to keep working for other reasons. For some women, work brings fulfillment and helps them define themselves. Or maybe work helps you to dwell on something other than the pain. Your job or career may be a treasured part of your life, a few hours every day when pain isn't your number-one focus. You get to interact with your work-family and to feel a part of the bigger world.

Hopefully your employer will be understanding and accommodating about your chronic condition. When considering what sorts of modifications you might require in order to continue doing your job, start by thinking about these questions:

- ◢ Can you afford to modify your full-time job to a part-time job?

- ◢ Can you take on fewer responsibilities?

- ◢ Can you change jobs inside your company to one that's easier?

- ◢ Can you work from home?

As is true with medical professionals, it helps to be proactive when dealing with an employer—that is, to approach your boss with a few well-considered options for accommodating your condition rather than waiting for her or him to come up with a plan. Your ideas can serve as a springboard from where you and your employers can start a dialogue about the situation, and your efforts will inspire their confidence that you have their interests at heart as well as your own.

In addition to whatever formal plan you develop with your employer, here are a few suggestions for living with FM at work:

◄ Take breaks from prolonged sitting and standing.

◄ Make sure your chair, desk, and work space are ergonomically correct.

◄ Lower your stress by being prepared and organized.

◄ Enlist your coworkers and your supervisors in brainstorming for ideas about how your work space can be modified to help you adjust to your job.

◄ Practice good boundaries. Break the habits of volunteering for overtime when you're exhausted and of taking on more work than you can reasonably finish in the time allotted.

Do everything in your power to make your job fit your needs. Think of all the ways in which you have taken the time to modify your house and your home life in order to coexist with FM. Do these things at work as well.

Denise P. Doing my job mostly keeps my mind off the pain during the day. My coworkers know about my illness, even if they don't understand what it means. They don't treat me any differently. My employer has provided accommodations for my illness. I got a new chair chosen especially to support my back; it is fully adjustable so I can relax and be comfortable. Before the new chair, I could hardly walk when I'd get up. I work a full forty-hour week unless I have to go in late or take a few hours off because of the pain, and I keep up with my own work. I am also able to volunteer for more work when people are on leave or we are short-staffed.

Sondra H. Some of my coworkers know of my condition. I don't think it's necessary for everyone to know. I try to keep my attitude up and blend in. People who are aware know when I'm having a rough day, though others may not. I still am able to perform well and to continue to grow at work. I pace myself carefully to manage my workload, but I continue to take on new challenges.

Working in my job, as an executive producer in television, has been a huge challenge. It's a business that is full of constant stresses and deadlines. The hours can be long at times. I've had to learn to manage that stress. There are some physical aspects of the business I cannot do any longer, but fortunately that is something I can work around. Many times I feel I have to alter my home life to be able to manage my career. In a two-income family, doing so is necessary. Does my family suffer? Not really; we've learned to adjust. It just means I may be unable to do certain activities, or I'll go to bed earlier. Also, if I can manage my workload, I have an understanding boss who allows me to take off early to adjust for the extra hours I work. But sometimes in this business that doesn't always happen. I can definitely feel when I've gone too hard at work; my FM never lets me slide.

Penny G. I need to help with the family income, but in the next two years I hope to cut back to part-time. I work an average of thirty-eight hours a week, with only Mondays off.

Most of my coworkers know about my illness, and some understand it. There have been no accommodations provided except some understanding when I say no to extra hours of work. Even with FM, I am very good at both of my jobs.

Ginger C. My coworkers know about my FM, and they know to let me do what I can and only to help me when I need it. I don't want to be treated differently. When I am feeling really bad, I like to get busy and distract myself with a project.

Rachel B. Being able to go to work every day makes my day, even if I have to rely on my wheelchair or cane at times. My work as an occupational therapy manager keeps me busy and makes me feel as if I'm still an active member of this community. That is really important to me. As my body lets me, I like to do as much physical activity as possible.

It's hard to explain to people—even to patients—why I sometimes have to rely on a cane or wheelchair to get around. Some patients seem to have more respect for me because I'm somewhat in the same boat as they are. They feel I am able to understand them better because I'm also disabled. Other people at work who also have a chronic condition have started to ask me more questions. They can talk to me about their problems and feel understood.

At times I feel scared about my job responsibilities. I have to rely on a body that sometimes can't withstand the physical demands of the job. During a flare-up, thoughts have crossed my mind saying, "What if...." Currently, whenever the physical aspect of my job is out of reach, I resort to hand therapy, massage therapy, ergonomics, and studying computer information management.

My coworkers know about my condition, although sometimes they are not fully aware of the limitations. I have to rely more on my staff to perform direct inpatient care. I take advantage of temporary accommodations whenever I need them. As long as I can do my job, I feel I make a positive contribution.

Sisu G. My immediate boss knows about my FM, and so does the woman whom I work with most. I work at a company with an in-house medical staff, and they, too, know. I don't keep it a secret from anyone. I got a few waves of pity as people found out, but mostly it doesn't change anything. I have to leave early from time to time, but that's it in terms of special accommodations. I do my job and it all works out. I'm still a very valuable part of the workforce. My bosses and coworkers don't know how much effort it is for me, and they probably won't. If I ever become crippled by this, at least my employers will have known from the beginning. There will never be any question of its being a surprise or a sudden medical claim. I intend to keep working, though. I like it here.

▲▲▲

FACING THE LOSS OF YOUR WORK

Often overlooked by healthy coworkers is the amount of preparation it takes for a chronically ill person to work an eight-hour-a-day job. If you have FM with IBS as a daily complication, for example, many days out of the month may be lost to diarrhea and the resulting dehydration, electrolyte imbalance, and exhaustion. Or if sleep is one of your biggest challenges, getting up and getting to work on time can be a problem. The list goes on. The difficulty lies not just in the ability to work for eight hours; some of us with FM could do that. It's in managing the surrounding hours before and after the workday.

Whether because of pain, fatigue, cognitive difficulties, or the stress of having a chronic illness, some women are disabled by FM and are forced to quit work. When your quality of life suffers because you are struggling too hard to maintain the delicate balance between work, taking good care of yourself, and keeping up with home and family, it may be time to leave your job and concentrate on healing. If your life consists only of working, eating, and sleeping, it has come to the point where you should consider making such a change. This is not an easy choice, especially if you are the sole wage earner in your household.

The majority of FM patients I speak with who have quit work miss their jobs and their work friends. The isolation represented by leaving the work world can be devastating. When life suddenly changes from a busy, thriving existence to one seemingly defined by frustrating pain and fatigue, we are left feeling sad, alone, and forgotten. I used to have a huge case of longing, a pressure-cooker urge to return to work. Just recently, I was able to let myself off the hook, refocus on my remission, and realize that being unable to work isn't going to break me. I can write a few hours a week as long as I rest and take care of myself, and for now that will have to be enough.

If you have left the work world, one of the challenges of living with FM is facing the inevitable question, "What do you do for a living?" Think in advance about how you will answer such an inquiry in a way that both informs the person asking and validates you. When I'm asked, I reply by saying, "I am unable to work as a florist right now because I am recovering from fibromyalgia and chronic fatigue syndrome."

It is an immense decision to quit your job, one the women whom we hear from below did not take lightly. They reported a responsibility to their employers and to their clients or patients—

and ultimately to themselves—when they made this life-changing choice.

Cybill C. I have been a registered nurse since I was twenty-three. My job is physically as well as mentally challenging. Last year, however, I had to stop working because I was unable to do my job. At the end, I was a danger to myself as well as to my patients. A simple mistake could kill someone, and my memory and cognitive skills diminished to the point where I couldn't even do a straightforward medical-dosage calculation. Nor did my employer like the fact that I frequently had to call in sick because I literally couldn't get out of bed. So I took a medical leave of absence.

Rae H. I am educated as a registered nurse (bachelor's degree level) and as a mental-health therapist (master's level). I worked all through my education, often full-time, and maintained a 3.9 GPA. It was difficult, but I had the energy to do it. When I first started working as a nurse and later as a social worker, I was required to do a great deal of multitasking. I thrived on it, loved the challenge. But as the years progressed, it became much more difficult to multitask. Gradually it has become so difficult that I am unable to think enough to put in a full eight-hour day. This is more bothersome than any other aspect of the FM—more frightening, more shameful, more demoralizing. I now work part-time as a therapist and three-quarters time on my book. I am frustrated by the length of time it takes to organize myself in relationship to the book and how much of my "housework" falls by the wayside, because I simply don't have enough clarity or energy to do it all. I do believe I am making positive contributions in my work and with my book, but I feel guilty about only working part-time.

The therapists with whom I consult and communicate in a professional capacity "know" about the FM, but they don't truly understand the extent and complexity of its limitations, because I don't connect with them on a prolonged, daily basis. As much as possible I am selective about when I initiate a phone call or a meeting. My last full-time job involved working with two male colleagues who didn't have a clue. My boss was a wonderful man, and as supportive as he could be, though he did not know about the FM. My coworker wasn't the kind of person I respected or felt "safe" around, with or without FM. The previous nursing job I had was a disaster, because the environment was noisy, the pace hectic, and the requirements for multitasking totally overwhelming. Each day was a nightmare.

FM has produced throat-clinching, heart-wrenching financial challenges. My inability to work full time impacts every corner of our world because of the financial stress placed on my husband. I am not receiving outside financial assistance. I have had clients who have struggled through the process of trying to get disability pay, and I don't have the courage or stamina to try to fight the system. It is my understanding that it is impossible to receive any kind of disability support if you are capable of working part-time. At this point in my life I would find it almost impossible to apply for that kind of assistance because I am still working part-time and because of the kind of work I do.

Katie G.   My life has changed radically since my diagnosis. For one thing, my physician ordered me to take a minimum of three months off from work. That alone changes anyone's life completely, especially a single woman's. I have a master's degree and had worked in computer sales in New York City, selling to major accounts such as Merrill Lynch, Colgate, Loews Corporation, and the New York Stock Exchange. In Seattle, with my current job, I covered seven states in computer network sales. I had devoted a great deal to my career and really enjoyed working. Once I was diagnosed, the major focus of my day was taken away because of my health. Like many Americans, I defined much of who I was by my job. Working provides so much more than money—the social interaction, the constant learning and exchanging of ideas, teamwork, personal goals and achievements, deadlines, project completions. Losing all of this created a void; I had to learn how to live a life with no predetermined structure, rules, goals, or paths.

American culture is achievement-oriented, status-conscious, and fast-paced. This illness is the antithesis of that. I've been told, "It's all in your head" (and actually some of it is—it's affected my brain capacity and function). It's difficult to go against the mainstream mentality and say, "No—my health and well-being are paramount." My priority is to take care of myself. Besides, I physically and mentally cannot do what I did prior to FM/CFS. I may stay at home, but I have the most challenging job of all—restoring my health. It is the most demanding job I have ever had.

Donnie M. I was fired from my job after my first surgery for TMJS because, as they put it, I had used up all my sick leave and vacation. They refused to let me have an hour off three times a week for physical therapy, which I had to undergo in order to get my mouth open due to scar-tissue buildup.

Gerry L. Going back to school and becoming an R.N. after raising my children was an accomplishment I was truly proud of. I excelled in my chosen profession. I was passionate about the responsibility I had taken on. I recognized that each patient was somebody's mother, grandmother, daughter, son, wife, or husband, not just "the GI bleed in room 721." I was truly a patient advocate. I had developed the instinct possessed by seasoned nurses.

The last nursing position I held was as a case manager in home-health nursing. That involved managing a caseload of patients and supervising ancillary services and looking after everything else that goes into being a nurse in the field on her own. Home-health nursing has developed into the ability to do almost anything that can be done in the hospital. It is high tech. It also involves terminal care.

I'm sure I had FM for a good part of my nursing practice. The last three to four years were a constant struggle, but I fought with all I had to continue. My home-health patients began to notice my fatigue, but their care was never compromised. I wouldn't stop until I'd done all I could for them, including interviews with doctors and insurance companies to get them what they needed.

I have priceless memories of the people I had the privilege to take care of. The difficult talks with family members. Sitting with a patient at three in the morning and offering emotional support because she had gotten bad news from her doctor earlier that night. I can't measure what the impact has been on me of discontinuing my work. Part of me is empty, gone, a void. Broken. My home-care supplies remain in the trunk of my car. My nurse's bag is still there. I can't empty it. I have tried many times. Not yet.

Diane H. I'm an attorney. The stress of my profession exacerbated my FM and forced me to leave my job. I've kept my license active by taking continuing legal-education courses, and although I haven't practiced in over two years, since we moved to southern Arizona, I'm finding other opportunities arising and other doors opening. If I continue to feel better, I expect to start a new business in the near future. When one door closes, another door opens. I truly feel that FM is part of the "plan" for my life and that I wouldn't have discovered these new opportunities if my illness hadn't pushed me in other directions.

Nancy D. FM caused me to lose my job. I have not worked since, and many doctors have told me not to expect to work. Irritable bowel syndrome kept me from being on time and kept me from my desk. My boss acted like I was slacking. Sleep problems were wearing me down quickly. I couldn't keep up. I was exhausted by the time I sat down at my desk in the morning. My coworkers knew only that my arms hurt. By the time I showered and dressed in the morning, my arms were throbbing with pain as if I'd been continuously holding a heavy tray.

I lost every workplace relationship I had. My employers, other than my immediate boss, were very accommodating, but I felt as if I had let everyone down. My situation had a heavy impact on the company. However, after all of the flowers and gifts I had ordered on behalf of my employer over the years, I felt undervalued because I didn't even receive a get-well card when I had almost lost the use of my arms for life. I think realistically they were just too busy to think about it. They did pack up my belongings and send them to my home via messenger, and they paid my medical insurance longer than necessary, mostly by accident, but they also terminated me thirty days sooner than they said they would.

Patricia S. I am a physician in a physically and mentally demanding field. With the onset of FM I'd start work at 7:00 A.M. and by 8:30 feel like I'd put in a whole day's work. It became impossible for me to work. I am not trained for a doctor's desk job, so that wasn't an option. My coworkers would not have had any sympathy for me if they knew. You either do your job or leave. There is no place for a permanently disabled worker. This attitude does not have any emotional value attached to it; it's an assembly line, and either you toe the line or step off the line. I miss the work, the self-esteem it gave me, and the knowledge that I was contributing to others' benefit. But I could not keep up to my standards, and sooner or later I feared I'd make a mistake that might be devastating to another person.

Now I am my number-one patient. But when I meet strangers whom I probably won't ever speak to again, I lie. I talk about my "job." I do not mention my illness. I do not like to discuss it with strangers. I also feel pressure from my boyfriend not to tell others about my illness. It's somewhat like mental illness. Don't talk about it in public. Keep it in the closet.

Jean T. When I first realized that my condition was serious, I was working as an interior designer. My boss told me they were going to lay me off because business was slow, and she felt that I was becoming too tired. I was tired, but I needed my job. I was devastated. I cried, and then I got angry and went out and got a much better job that paid more and involved less heavy lifting. Then I decided to get my real estate license and work closer to home. I could control my hours better and be with my husband more. I quit working altogether a year and a half before he passed away. I made that decision as much as a result of my illness as his.

I experienced some very frightening incidents while working in real estate. One Sunday when I was at an open house, it snowed about a foot. When it came time to go home, I walked out the door to the top of fifteen steps that didn't have a handrail. Because of my lack of balance, I was afraid I would fall, so I threw my briefcase to the ground, sat down, and slid to the bottom. At least I didn't fall. (I was pretty wet and cold, though.) It wasn't long afterward that I gave up work entirely. Putting out signs got to be too much of a high-wire act to suit me. My balance was so far gone and I was in so much pain that I had a hard time doing what I had to do. When someone once suggested that I had been drinking, I knew it was time to give it up.

Victoria M. I have not worked for five years now, and although I miss the money, companionship, and a change from being at home, it is not an option for me to return to the workplace. I previously worked in a pharmacy and trained as a florist just before I collapsed. I cannot stand for long periods of time, which my work entailed, or carry heavy boxes, etc. I am chemically sensitive, and bright lights and loud noises are still a bother for me.

I plan to study psychology and philosophy, and would like to establish a clinic for diagnosis and treatment of FM/CFS patients. Support and counseling are imperative for these patients and their families and friends. I feel well-situated from my personal experiences to embark on such a journey. Presently, however, my family needs my support and I am still recovering. I will not entertain the idea of working at the types of jobs I have had before. I would like to be my own boss, pursue what I believe in, and develop something the community will benefit from. FM and CFS have changed my career directions!

Although I am not in the workforce as such, I believe I am making positive contributions which satisfy my need to belong and be useful. Although the money is handy, I think people forget or are unaware that work is not the be-all and end-all. I think there is too much emphasis placed on what you do rather than who you are.

Marcia D. I was cooking at one of the local high schools, which is really a high-stress job. You have only so much time to do things, and there's a lot of lifting. I think if I had felt better I probably would have continued to thrive and done quite well. But it got to the point about four years ago where I finally had to quit because I couldn't do it anymore. I would go to work and have to come home and take pain pills, and it was kind of a Catch-22.

I've thought about going back to work. Mentally, I think it would be good for me. My biggest fear is wondering who would hire me when I can't use my hands. And since I take narcotic pain medication, I don't think anyone is going to look at me and say, "You're hired."

▲▲▲

If you are unable to work or have had to change jobs because of FM, consider the following: Your expectations of a full life do not have to fit into society's view of the "norm," so don't let your job define you. You are so much more than the title on your desk, nameplate, or punch card. If there are insurmountable pressures within your job, realize that such a situation does the illness no good.

Also recognize that a job doesn't always mean forty hours of work outside the home. If in order to save your health you must cut back on your hours or find creative ways to occupy yourself from home, do so without looking back. Your number-one task is to take care of yourself and to heal. The job you do to make money should support that end.

Think of yourself and your family, and be sure you all come out on top.

LETTING GO OF GUILT AND PRESSURE

I have a pass that allows me to park in a handicapped space. It also allows me to park free at a parking meter. Just like many other people with an invisible disability, when I've availed myself of these benefits, I've sometimes been confronted by "helpful" folks pointing out that I am parked in a handicapped spot. I have used the pass to park in a space marked for disabled people only about four times in the last nine years. Usually I'll drive around looking for a regular spot that is close by, because I know that folks who use wheelchairs need the wider space. I do use the pass downtown, where my doctor's office is located, to park at a meter within a few blocks of his office. Some days I don't go to the store because of the amount of walking required, both in the store and in the parking lot. Ninety-nine percent of the time, I am able to walk any reasonable distance from the parking lot to the store, because I only shop on good days. That's the thing with FM, inconsistency. Some days you have bone-crushing fatigue and some days you can walk a few blocks.

Because sometimes I can walk across a parking lot, several thoughts used to go through my mind when I used the parking pass. Am I disabled *enough*? Do I really qualify? These questions came up for me recently when I was at a government office. A disabled man worked behind the counter. He seemed to have limited use of one arm, and he used a wheelchair to move around the office. Seeing his more obvious disability reminded me that I have had to let go of guilt over whether or not I "qualify" as disabled.

Now, however, I have the inner knowledge that I am being responsible and honest when I use my parking pass, and I no longer worry about it.

I've made the decision to draw the line at calling myself *disabled*. I formerly used the term but eventually felt that I limited myself in doing so. Now I choose the attitude that I have a chronic-pain condition that keeps me from working a steady, regular job. Does that mean my friends who use a cane, walker, oxygen tank, or wheelchair are more accepted as legitimately "disabled"? Unfortunately, in our society, yes.

What is the best way to handle questions about our health? Depending on who is asking, I usually explain what FM is and isn't, and let it go at that. If it is a person I have just met, I will likely spend a moment discussing FM with them. More often than not, strangers nowadays seem to know someone with FM. Countless times I have met someone whose family member has FM. I constantly give out my card and talk to people I have just met. I know that every person I educate about FM will benefit someone else down the line.

Why am I telling you this? Because I spent an awful lot of time worrying and wondering about what people thought of my illness, the fact that I couldn't work, and the fact that my partner had to take care of me at times. What brought this time-wasting game to a halt was when someone told me plainly that for the most part, *people just don't care!* What? Neighbors aren't spending their days wondering if I'm faking? People I only recently met aren't thinking less of me because we live off my partner's income?

In the beginning of my new life with FM, I wanted everyone to know why I was not working. I felt that if I could just explain FM to them, I could somehow deal with all of my own unanswered questions as well. I believed incorrectly that my neighbors thought I was faking the severity of my illness when I could go outside and pull weeds or work in my front garden for a half hour.

In truth, they saw me for what I was at the time, scared, fatigued, and in pain. One neighbor told me that they used to watch me get in and out of my truck and limp up the stairs, and they felt sad. I never knew this. Being open from the beginning with my wonderful neighbors and friends would have freed me from a year of anxiety. Here's the lesson I learned from this: Don't spend your precious energy worrying about what other people may or may not believe.

I hope you hear in what I am saying that it is up to you to decide how you will represent your invisible illness. Will you take people's hard admonitions to heart? Or will you make it a goal to educate people about your illness and then let it go and get on with learning to live well?

Money Matters: Paying the Bills and Getting the Benefits We're Entitled To

Losing our income and lifestyle are two of the greatest difficulties of living with a serious chronic illness such as fibromyalgia. FM is different from most other types of illness or disability in that it affects so many of our body's systems and therefore prohibits us from working at jobs that other disabled individuals can manage, such as security guard or video monitor, two jobs I have seen listed as possibilities in Social Security denial letters. The officials who compose such letters fail to understand that having FM prevents us from being able to sit or stand for long periods and that fatigue is always in the forefront.

So what will you do if FM keeps you from working at any job whatsoever? How in the world will you survive, especially if you're single? First of all, try to prevent your fearful thoughts from spiraling into panic. Many resources exist for those who've lost the security of a regular paycheck due to disability, but tapping into them can require single-mindedness and persistence. It's natural to feel worried under circumstances like these, but you can't afford to waste your energy fueling the worst-case scenarios that may pop into your mind. Recognize any fear that comes up, and then move ahead to focusing on solution-oriented thinking—and read this chapter carefully for guidance and support.

MEETING BASIC NEEDS

I am thankful I had a home, a partner, and parents to support me when I had to give up my job. Otherwise, although good social services are available in Seattle, I don't know what I would have done to stay afloat. I have watched friends move into group homes, exhaust their savings, loot their IRAs, get on lists for public housing, and go to food banks. Around the time I lost my job, I heard a radio program about poverty. The narrator talked about getting extra money by selling off high-ticket items like boats and campers, holding garage sales, even living in your car if you exhaust your funds. It's true that FM can steal everything you own, but most of us have family and friends who wouldn't let us starve or end up homeless.

The best thing to do if it looks like you'll have to quit working is to *get organized*. Start by making a list of the most pressing things you need, such as:

◀ Money

◀ Rent/housing

◀ Food

◀ Child care

◀ Help with taking care of your home

◀ Transportation to doctors' offices

Next, call every social-service agency that might be able to help you. If you cannot do this because of fatigue, pain, or cognitive difficulties, ask a friend to lend a hand with making phone calls. Keep on calling until you get assistance with obtaining welfare, food, health-care coupons, or with contacting the agencies you need.

If you have lost your job because of FM, don't waste any time signing up for short-term assistance. Call your state's social-services department right away. It can assist you with signing up for welfare while waiting for your Social Security benefits to be awarded.

Your state's social-services department (called the Department of Social and Health Services, or DSHS, in the state of Washington) may assign a case manager to assist you. This is valuable. He or she can help you apply for Social Security benefits and navigate the rest of the social services out there. Doing so can be very time-consuming and confusing, especially if you haven't needed to use the services before, so it's useful to have an expert guide.

If you are a member of a church, synagogue, or mosque, let your fellow worshippers know of your condition. Many of my friends have been helped this way. Even if you aren't a member, call a local church and ask if sponsorship is available, or ask friends or relatives to call theirs. There are also agencies, sometimes utilizing the help of volunteers, that can help you clean your house and run errands.

Do not be ashamed to ask for help from friends and family. I have found that friends want to help but don't know what to do. They are often grateful to be "given an assignment," so to speak. Everyone in my support group has helped one another at different times. Whether it was with moving, transportation to appointments, or even cooking, we stood behind each other in the early days of our illness. One time my group raised money, bought presents, and put together an entire Christmas dinner for an ill woman and her children. My group was the catalyst, and healthy people made it happen. It is truly amazing what can be accomplished when you just ask folks for their support. People are very generous.

Sisu G. I made twenty-five thousand dollars in the year 2001. My medical bills totaled more than twenty thousand dollars. I was without insurance and without answers until November. One week I spent my whole paycheck on medications. The medications didn't work, and I didn't know what to do. The hospitals ended up giving me free care, which covered the worst of the bills. But I was scared.

When you're at the bottom of the ladder, you realize that if something bad happens to you and you can't work, you're screwed. There is no safety net. There's no immediate disability pay, and if you can't pay your rent, you're out on the street. I was lucky; I was living with a friend. If I hadn't been, then what?

Medical care is in a state of crisis in this country, and those with chronic illness who can't work are the ones who don't have it and yet who need it the most. Nobody's quite sure what to do about it, but everyone agrees that something must be done. I was lucky, that's all. Every time I pass a homeless person I think about what it would have been like to have been out on the street with this disease. Not everyone has a friend or a family to take them in. I wonder what's wrong with this picture, that disability carries such a stigma.

Gina H. I am not working. We have lost our savings, the money we had set aside for our son's college education. We have asked for food stamps and were denied because they said my husband made too much. How can we make too much and be unable to afford medication? We had to use our credit cards to pay bills. Now we are seeking help from Consumer Credit Counseling. I had to stop going to my therapist once a week because we could not afford that. We are trying to make it from week to week. I feel so bad; I feel this is my fault because of this illness.

Emma L. Because my earnings dropped, I have spent almost half of my IRA to meet financial needs.

Sondra H. There have definitely been times of financial challenge. The medications are not cheap, and when we were trying to find the right medications, we went through a lot of money. The pain-clinic treatment was another huge expense that made things financially tight for my family. And even now, with trying to keep my muscles limber and to avoid knots where they inject medications, I incur the cost of massages twice a month (I actually should be going once a week). It is a financial commitment my family has to assume.

Cybill C. It is very financially challenging to have FM. Since I cannot work, I have to rely on other sources of income to make ends meet. I take so many medications that my copayments really added up. I found myself taking medications every other day to make them last longer because I simply couldn't afford taking them daily.

My major life stressor is financial. It is hard to be on the brink of poverty. I deal with it by doing free things with my kids, such as trips to the zoo or park. I tell myself that my children can still be happy and healthy without a lot of money.

Victoria M. We have had a dreadful time with social services—the system rather than the individuals in it. The social-service system in Australia does not recognize FM as a long-term, disabling illnesses. They do not ask the correct questions in order to appreciate the type of disabilities suffered. We cannot diagnostically prove our pain or fatigue. I have been told that I need to approach my politician to have the criteria changed in order for patients to get help. The powers-that-be seem to think you are a lesser person. The battle is not worth the suffering endured. I have trouble dealing with people who are close-minded and write off everything to the system and its failings.

The financial situation has been harrowing. The endless costs of my medical consultations, tests, treatments (which offer no guarantees), and the loss of my income together with my engineer husband's being out of work twice in the past four years has been very, very stressful. The specific food requirements are expensive. We have used all our savings and most of our retirement. We cannot pay off our home; we are currently making interest payments only. We are managing to educate our children and pay their expenses. They are not well enough to work and study.

APPLYING FOR SOCIAL SECURITY BENEFITS

Making the decision to apply for Social Security benefits is a big step and can be very difficult for some women to come to terms

with. The label of *disabled person* is tough to accept if you have
been healthy your whole life. I have known people who have
waited for years to apply for SS, slipping further and further into
poverty, unable to admit that FM has taken away their ability to
work.

Before you begin, call the Social Security Administration (find
the toll-free phone number below or in Resources) and ask for the
pamphlet titled *Basic Facts about Social Security*. It contains all
the information you need to know to apply for benefits. Knowing
what to expect will help you be less apprehensive. With the
mounds of paperwork to fill out and the multitiered process
involved, applying for Social Security benefits can feel like walking
through a maze. But really, dealing with the Social Security
Administration just takes knowledge, patience, and time to navigate your way through the steps. After all, remember that the benefits are yours. You've paid into the system.

Also be aware that the sooner you sign up for Social Security
benefits, the larger your award will be, because they determine
your monthly payment by the wages you have earned in the past.
This is called *earned income credits*. As soon as you qualify for benefits, you will receive a monthly check that is determined by your
past wages, and you will also qualify for Medicare insurance.

When you apply for benefits, the Social Security Administration will tell you if you qualify for Social Security Disability (SSD)
or Supplemental Security Income (SSI). To qualify for SSD, you
must have been disabled by your illness for twelve months and
have worked long enough before applying to earn enough income
credits, including five of the last ten years. SSI is a federally
funded program for people who are disabled and also low income.
To qualify, you don't need earned income credits.

As soon as you are ready to begin, contact your local Social
Security office (call toll free [800] 772-1213 to find the office nearest you). Or visit the Social Security Administration website at
www.ssa.gov. By calling Social Security or visiting the website you
can learn more about these programs, along with determining the
amount of benefits you qualify for. And as of January 2002, you

can apply for Social Security benefits online at the above-mentioned website, or you can apply by phone. This may make it easier for those who are too ill to drive to an office. If you have cognitive difficulties and find the long forms confusing, ask for help from a friend or case manager.

It's best to get started on the paperwork right away because the process takes a long time. There are several illnesses for which people are automatically awarded benefits after applying, such as forms of terminal cancer. Everyone else has to go through the system level by level. It's a lengthy and tedious process of applications, hearings, and appeals.

Luckily, in April 1999, the Social Security Administration issued Ruling 99-2p, which officially recognized that FM and CFS are "medically determinable impairments." This answers the question of whether a person with FM can be awarded benefits. Ruling 99-2p uses the diagnostic criteria from the Centers for Disease Control and Prevention and the American College of Rheumatology. Now, as with every other illness or impairment, people with FM are judged on an individual basis.

You may already have a case manager if you have applied for state assistance. In Washington, if you apply for welfare or GAU (Government Assistance for the Unemployable), you are automatically signed up to begin the Social Security application process.

Gina H. We are not receiving any assistance. It took a long time for me to admit we needed help. Now I have a lawyer trying to help me get SSI. It was very hard to ask for help. I can remember when I went to the Social Security office and looked at the other people there. I thought, "What am I doing here?" The other folks looked like they needed help more than I did. But I held my head high and filled out those papers, hoping that we will get some kind of help. We were denied twice. That is the thing: FM patients don't look sick, so they just turned their noses up at me. Very rude people. Now we have bill collectors calling. They are really stressing me out.

Gerry L. I do receive SS disability benefits. I took no legal action. It took over six months of hard work, a lot of it done from my bed.

The process was so overwhelming that it seems clearly designed to encourage people to give up. I can't imagine someone who's alone, sick, and/or elderly getting through it without assistance. It was a unique and most unpleasant experience. I will say that the people I dealt with, one of whom was my adjudicator, were courteous and kind. I was tenacious. I kept good chronological records. Was it hard to admit I needed help? You bet!!! It is not part of my work ethic. You work for what you earn. Yet I had contributed to SS all the years I worked and therefore was eligible.

I was awarded on first try, which is quite unusual for someone with fibromyalgia, from what I've read and heard. When I started the process, one of the first staffers I talked to told me that if I had applied three years earlier, when I'd stopped working, I would have received more money. She made this comment after looking through my information and noticing a big drop in my wages. I was very thorough and documented everything. I gave them all the information they asked for and was very specific in my answers. Having to provide the kind of details they wanted was not pleasant, but I answered each question honestly. I even sent along copies of my job descriptions from all of the positions I'd held. I think they were a bit overwhelmed.

I saw two doctors, at their request, which was the most inhumane and demeaning part of the process. What an eye-opener. I asked each one if I could tape-record the visit. They both refused. It was an assembly-line moneymaker for them. The first one, an internist, knew little to nothing about FM. That was one of my questions for him. I had given better assessments to patients than he did to me. He didn't know where to start. They had a very big problem getting him to file his report. The other doctor was a psychiatrist. Each had a standardized questionnaire to follow. I believe without it they wouldn't have known what to ask. I was polite but confident. When asked if I was ever depressed, I replied, "If you could no longer sit behind your desk and do what you are doing because of a life-changing event, wouldn't you feel sad or depressed?" He answered yes. So did I. And on it went. But before I left, I explained to him that FM was like being on a battlefield waiting for the shot to be fired, not knowing when it would hit or how bad it would be. And I emphasized that the pain was in my body, not my head. He gave me his card and told me to see a psychiatrist and take an antidepressant. I thanked him for his suggestion and left. What a joke.

Afterward I asked, "Why send me to doctors who know very little about FM?" The Social Security Administration told me it would cost too much to send patients to specialists. My case was referred for review to its own panel of doctors, who seemed to have trouble making a decision. They asked my permission for one of their doctors to speak to my rheumatologist, something I had suggested before. Now they wanted to talk to the expert on FM who knew my condition. They had already received a written report from him and also one from my counselor. Still, I gladly gave them permission to speak to my doctor.

In the end I received a lump sum dating back a year. I now receive a monthly check. It felt very strange at first, but I'm getting used to it.

Carol J. The financial challenges are overwhelming. I went from a $40,000 joint business income to $580 per month on disability.

I receive both Social Security Disability and SSI, which takes care of all my medical and prescription-drug expenses, teeth, and eyeglasses. It was very difficult to finally admit that I could no longer be self-supportive and independent and gainfully employed. But since I did work for thirty-three years, I figured I paid into the system, so it is acceptable to receive something in compensation.

Jean T. I did have financial challenges. I was sixty-two when I started receiving Social Security benefits. My husband was five years older than I, so he had been getting benefits for some time. Receiving his monthly check was great, but it was not enough for us to make it very comfortably. Yet somehow, we did.

I am getting other financial assistance as well. I receive coverage from Medicaid for my prescriptions, which would cost over nine hundred dollars per month otherwise. I am in a federal program known as COPES, which is administered by the state. Its aim is to help people stay out of nursing homes. They help me get assistance with my everyday chores.

I did not know that I would be eligible to receive my husband's Social Security benefits once he died. I was afraid I would have to become a bag lady. My own Social Security payment was hardly adequate to buy food. I am so grateful. I have a beautiful apartment, my car, and enough money to live a comfortable life. I believe God has his angels looking after me. It could not have worked out better for me; if only I didn't have this illness, life would be perfect. I did not have to take legal action, thank goodness. I suppose it was because of our age. We were undoubtedly eligible. It was and is hard to admit and ask for help.

My goals are different now from what they once were. I grew older faster than I ever planned to. I planned on both of us working at least another fifteen to twenty years and then on traveling and generally having fun.

Katie G. My financial challenges boil down to going from an excellent full-time sales job with numerous benefits (i.e., health insurance, 401K, stock options) to fighting for two and a half years to get Social Security Disability. It was quite scary and I ran through much of my savings. I live frugally and am told that I may never be able to qualify for a mortgage because I do not have an income.

I am receiving Social Security Disability benefits and had to hire a lawyer to make it happen. I took out a small, private disability policy on myself when I was in my late twenties and also currently receive payments from that. I fought for my disability insurance and at first was shocked to be applying for Social Security. I refused to be on Medicare as a thirty-five-year-old. Psychologically, it was too much, so I pay for my own health insurance each month.

I have been most fortunate because my professional jobs allowed me to save and invest money for this life emergency.

Donna P. I have gone from riches to poverty. I am on Social Security Disability and that is my only income. Thank heavens my home and car are paid for, or I would be living on the streets.

Marcia D. I never even thought about disability when I stopped working. I figured after a few months off I would go back to work. Not! Since I'm unable to use my hands and arms like most people, I soon realized that no one would hire me. So I started the long process with Social Security.

My doctor was great about working with me. He sent all of my records to Social Security, along with three years of records from my shrink. My doctor stated that I was unable to work and that he saw this as a long-term illness. All my papers were reviewed by Social Security and I was sent to a Social Security doctor, who spent ten minutes with me and decided that I was able to work.

I didn't have the energy to go back and fight with them after I received that decision. I don't know how they can spend ten minutes with a person and decide that she is eligible to work, when I've had the same doctor for twenty to thirty years and he knows me better than anyone.

Cybill C. I am currently receiving welfare while waiting for my Social Security Disability claim to be approved. I applied in March of 2001 and have not yet received a determination. If I am denied, I will seek a lawyer to gain approval.

When to Hire an Attorney

If you have been denied your Social Security benefits on the first try, you mustn't give in to discouragement. Most people get turned down on the first go-around. In fact, I know of only a few people who were awarded benefits without having to reapply.

Now you enter the phase called *reconsideration*. This is generally the best time to get an attorney involved. Find one who will work up front for you. He or she will get paid only if you win; you will pay him or her a percentage of the award you receive from Social Security.

Alternatively, some firms offer nonattorney legal representation for people seeking to claim Social Security benefits. Disability Advocates, based in Sacramento, California, is one such organization (see in Resources under "Websites").

You and your attorney (or other representative) will discuss your case and decide on the appropriate time frame for legal representation. The Social Security Administration gives an applicant sixty days to reapply for reconsideration. At this stage, another round of paperwork is required, including an activity form, a pain-and-fatigue form, and a typical-day form. Again, be very thorough in filling out the paperwork. It does you no good to hold back. You must admit the truth of your situation, no matter how grim. Be up-front in letting them know about your pain levels and the amount of fatigue you endure. Your candor and openness will give SS a good idea of the severity of your illness and of what your days are like.

The Hearing

If your claim is rejected during the reconsideration phase, again, don't be discouraged. This is fairly common. You can appeal the decision by asking for a hearing. Many people win their cases at hearings. In fact, it was at their hearings that most of the women I spoke with were awarded their benefits. You must ask for a hearing in writing within sixty days of the date your reconsideration is denied.

The hearing will take place in front of an administrative law judge. It is a closed hearing—just you, a support person if you choose, your attorney or other legal representative, a stenographer, and the judge. On Social Security's behalf, there may be one or more "witnesses" testifying against you or simply against the possibility of your having FM. There may also be witnesses testifying on your behalf.

Before the hearing you may be examined by a doctor working for the Social Security Administration or by a psychiatrist. It is very important to take notes along to these visits to help you remember dates, medications, and important facts. Stick to the facts. Try to view these professionals as you would one of your doctors. Be up-front and open about your condition. However, remember that these doctors may be biased, and they may know nothing about FM. Keep a cool head, inform them well about your condition, but don't expect much. This visit is purely investigational by the Disability Determination Service and the doctors and psychiatrists who work for the SSA.

It is important to be prepared for your hearing. (Your attorney or legal representative will help you with this; it's a large part of what they are paid to do.) Ask your friends and coworkers to write letters testifying to the fact that you are ill. It's best to have letters from people who knew you before you became ill so that they can write about the changes they have seen in your health. Your attorney will also ask for letters from members of your health-care team. These lend a lot of weight.

Make sure the records you present from your primary-care physician are impeccable. Be sure he has precisely recorded your pain and fatigue levels on each visit, your painful tender points, your medications, and every other little fact that might help you get the benefits you deserve. Be sure also that his statement says you are disabled.

Nancy D.   I've experienced every financial challenge imaginable. I lost my job, my health insurance, a third of my income, my life-insurance policy, my apartment in the city, and can contribute nothing to my 401K plan. My professional wardrobe is now useless; it had to be completely replaced by cotton and loose-fitting clothes. I live in pajamas a lot.

My condition started as a worker's comp injury, and that insurance company was the most difficult to work with. They required many reports from my doctor and held back treatments requested by my doctor, and then they cut me off for financial benefits after some time, without notice. Once I figured out what happened, I had to scramble to apply for state disability. That claim got lost and had to be completely resubmitted, which involved more waiting.

My employer provided a long-term disability (LTD) policy that paid out a small sum after ninety days of disability. My claim was to be completed by me and my doctor and submitted to the LTD insurance company. My employer inadvertently filed away the paperwork. After waiting a long time, I called the LTD insurance company and was informed that my employer had not submitted the claim. My employer was on vacation. It got resolved, but it took many more weeks.

I went to an FM support-group meeting that featured as a speaker an attorney specializing in Social Security. He discussed the entire application process. When I moved to Washington, I called him, and he referred me to a fabulous attorney in Seattle who specializes in FM/CFS claims. I had already been denied twice, and it was only after the hearing in front of a judge with my attorney that I was granted SSI and Medicare benefits. It took two years, but I finally did win SSI benefits.

▲▲▲

As you can see, applying for Social Security benefits requires lots of patience, time, and effort. If your claim is still denied after the hearing, the next step is the Appeals Council. Then, if your case is still unsuccessful, it's on to the U.S. District Court.

PRIVATE INSURANCE

Sometimes paying for private disability insurance through your employer doesn't work out the way you thought it would. You believe that the insurance will be there for you if something happens and you need it, but many respondents to my survey have learned otherwise. People have told me that private insurance companies go to great lengths to make it difficult for claimants to receive benefits. Or they pay out for a while and then find a clause "justifying" a termination of benefits.

Just as with Social Security, when dealing with a private insurer, you must prove that you are disabled and that you continue to stay disabled. Keeping good records is a must, and so is making sure that your doctor takes time to document your case completely.

Below, the women share about their experiences with private disability insurers. They also discuss the financial repercussions of their medical insurance—such as covering out-of-pocket costs and expensive copayments.

Cydney B. It's depressing to think of the loss of my six-figure-a-year job and of my having to cash in stock options that today would be worth literally millions.

I have received Social Security Disability since I became eligible in February 1995, six months after I left my job. I have undergone two medical examinations for Social Security since then. My benefits were terminated once, but after we filed other reports with the SSA, they were reinstated.

I was so fortunate (I thought) to have the "Cadillac" of LTD plans at the time I left my employment at the biotech company. Being a health-care company, they made sure their benefits package was the best. I was insured for disability payments for as long as I was unable to perform "all the essential requirements" of the exact job I held when I left work because of my illness. That meant I had to be able to return to an associate-director-level job in a large company, or they had to pay my benefits until I was sixty-five years old.

In 1997, the insurance company sent me to their doctor, who said I didn't have rheumatoid arthritis, didn't have FM, and was a psychiatric case. This was a classic LTD strategy of cutting off benefits to those insured under Cadillac policies, and as a human-resources professional I knew it full well. I'd seen it happen to a lot of other people. I got a lawyer. I went to the Mayo Clinic on my own dollar, and after six months of wrangling, the insurance company reinstated my benefits prior to our filing any court action. However, I accepted a lower level of benefits, so my husband had to return to work (he had retired in 1996).

Since his full retirement in 2000, we have a lower income, but we are very comfortable. Other factors outside my illness allowed us to have a comfortable retirement. Still, disability payments are part of our income.

Lalenya R. My disability forced me to leave a very good-paying position as a marketing director. Fortunately my husband makes a good living. I am still unemployed.

For the first two years, I received employer-paid disability, then the insurer cut off my benefits. Currently, we are in a lawsuit about the "self-reported clause" that many disability insurers have snuck into their contracts in order to avoid paying for FM, CFS, Gulf War Syndrome, and myriad other diseases. Because most group disability contracts are covered under ERISA, no punitive damages are allowed and hence few attorneys want to take your case. I'll be lucky to get any part of my benefits reinstated, and if I do, the lawyer will take 33 percent of it.

Marcia D. When my husband's company changed insurance carriers, the copay for prescriptions went up enormously. Out of our own pocket, we pay four hundred dollars per month for my medications. The copayments for name-brand drugs are high, and only a few of the drugs I take are generic.

Val T. Our insurance has paid well for my doctor visits and treatments. This year was the first year we spent the maximum out-of-pocket expense, so now we have 100 percent coverage until the first of next year. I have continued to work, so we have not suffered any financial loss other than the out-of-pocket expense (20 percent) required by the insurance plan. Prescriptions are covered, with a copayment of five dollars for generic drugs and fifteen dollars for nongenerics.

I receive no governmental assistance for FM and have absolutely no plans of ever doing so! I could not handle being at home, as I need to stay active to control the pain. I notice when I'm sedentary for a couple days. I always pay for it. I will never give up the fight. Doing so would be the end of me.

If you have already made the difficult decision to apply for government-sponsored benefits, whether through your state's welfare system or through Social Security, my advice is to hang in there. You are in for a long fight. The system is set up to make benefits available only to those who truly qualify. If you are disabled, keep on fighting for the benefits to which you are entitled. Remember, you have paid into Social Security all of your working life. If you need to take advantage of those benefits, it is up to you to be persistent and to represent the state of your illness to the best of your ability.

Never give up. Securing disability benefits is one of the most important parts of your treatment process. Once you ensure them, you can concentrate on doing everything possible to feel better.

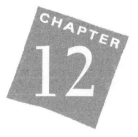

What's New? What's Coming?

In this chapter, which discusses some of the ongoing developments in both conventional medicine and complementary therapies, I let a handful of experts do most of the talking. You'll read about one physician's approach to treating fibromyalgia with prescription drugs, about some of the latest clinical research being conducted on FM, and about two "alternative" therapies that explore innovative angles for treating FM.

A PHARMACOLOGICAL APPROACH

Christopher Lawrence, M.D., has been a board-certified neurologist since 1984. He's in practice in Seattle. Here he tells us about his method of treating FM with prescription medicines:

▲▲▲

Few neurologists have an interest in fibromyalgia. I became interested in it twelve or thirteen years ago when I started working with soft-tissue body workers and naturopaths who referred fibromyalgia patients to me. We don't know exactly what fibromyalgia is. I define it as a group of diseases of chronic muscle pain associated with a decrease in deep sleep, feelings of fatigue, and interference with the quality of people's lives. Any number of conditions fit into that category; they don't necessarily have to meet the American College of Rheumatology guidelines for FM. People report pain differently. I have some patients who have been told by rheumatologists that they don't have fibromyalgia, but when they come to me, I say, "I don't care what you have; we'll just treat it as if you have fibromyalgia"—and they do fine on my regimen. I think a whole group of people exists who because of the way they report pain may not meet the formal criteria for FM, that is, pain in all four quadrants of the body, plus eleven out of eighteen tender points.

Fibromyalgia's cluster of disorders usually results in a vicious cycle. People either are injured, have a viral illness, or something else happens, and then their sleep becomes disrupted, and they become less active physically; therefore, they lose aerobic conditioning, so they cut back further on their exercise, they sleep poorly, and on and on. The key part of treatment is to figure out some combination of medicines that helps to normalize the patient's neurochemistry so they can get deep sleep or feel better during sleep and thus wake up rested so they can be more physically active. Because some of my early patients didn't want to take prescription medicines, I began experimenting with microscopic doses.

I have found that many patients need three or four medicines, but in very low doses. It doesn't seem as though any one medicine offers the real cure, and it seems as though a lot of fibromyalgia patients cannot tolerate regular dosages of traditional medicines. They have to start at almost homeopathic levels and gradually build up. It is a slow process. Patients usually take minimum doses for a year or two. At that point, if they are able to engage in both aerobic and stretching exercises, such as tai chi or yoga, and if they are managing the stress in their life, then we try to get them off medications. Another reason we combine medications is to balance the drugs' side effects.

Antidepressants and Muscle Relaxants

Typical drug combinations to treat FM include an antidepressant, which can treat pain, sleep disturbance, and depression. It may be an SSRI (selective serotonin reuptake inhibitor), or perhaps Wellbutrin, mirtazapine (Remeron), Effexor, or Serzone. It could be any one of the antidepressants, depending on the symptoms.

If a patient is terribly fatigued, I may prescribe Prozac in a very low dose. (About 20 to 30 percent of fibromyalgia patients cannot tolerate the generic version of Prozac; they are too sensitive to the generic's dosage fluctuations.) Zoloft also works pretty well; however, a lot of women complain about its sexual side effects. These patients seem to tolerate Celexa somewhat better.

Many people with fibromyalgia also suffer from clenching, or neck and jaw tension. Only a few medicines address this problem. The antianxiety med BuSpar is one that does, but taken alone it doesn't seem to work. Therefore, patients must take it in combination with one of the other neurotransmitter enhancers, either an SSRI or Wellbutrin or another antidepressant.

The dose of BuSpar required to treat clenching is often far less than that needed to treat anxiety. For example, the typical dose for anxiety is 30 mg (milligrams) a day. By contrast, I typically start people on one-fourth of a 5-mg tablet, or 1 mg. Most people get relief from clenching on a nighttime dose between 2.5 mg and 5 mg, but some patients can't even tolerate a dose that low, because they experience side effects such as nightmares, agitated sleep, or feeling too drugged the next day. On the other hand, if they have a prominent anxiety component, then I increase the BuSpar to a full dose over the course of a few months. That helps the anxiety, and it also helps the antidepressant work better. The same principle applies with the antidepressant; we often start at one-fourth of a small-dose pill and gradually build up. If the patient has a true depressive component, then they need a full dose. If they have just the myofascial pain and the fibromyalgia, then we can get by with a lower dose.

Since many people with fibromyalgia also suffer from restless-legs syndrome, if a patient cannot tolerate BuSpar, then I'll try a medicine like Mirapex. Developed for Parkinson's disease, Mirapex works in FM patients to treat restless legs, and it also helps clenching.

The other medicine that sometimes works for clenching is magnesium. Some European studies show that magnesium supplementation up to 750 mg daily over six or eight weeks can help clenching, but my experience with it so far shows its effects to be relatively mild. Some people in the United States believe that certain forms of magnesium are better than others; I am still experimenting with different forms to see if that holds true.

Typically, SSRIs work well for people who suffer tendonitis due to overuse of their arms or forearms; this class of medicines tends to relax the upper trapezius (the muscle along the back of the neck, shoulder, and upper back), as well as other muscles.

I can tell from a patient's pattern of muscle tightness which class of medicines they need. Each type of medicine seems to relax certain muscle groups better than others. BuSpar works best on the clenching muscles, which include the masseters (in the jaw), the scalenes (running from the neck vertebrae to the first and second ribs), the sternocleidomastoid (a long neck muscle running to the breastbone and collarbone), the thoracic paraspinals (between the shoulder blades), the psoas (hip flexors), the deep hamstrings, and the foot muscles. A lot of people who suffer from clenching also get plantar fasciitis, which is inflammation of the fascia in the sole of the foot. That group of muscles seems to respond best to BuSpar, and when one group starts to relax, the others follow. If they all relax except the clenching muscles, then I know there may be something wrong with the jaw, and that's when I get a TMJ (temporomandibular joint) practitioner involved. I usually don't get a TMJ practitioner involved until the rest of the muscles are looser and we know there is nothing else we can do chemically.

Besides assessing muscle tightness to determine which drugs a patient needs, I also use this method to determine dosage. For example, if at six weeks I see that a patient's forearms and anterior chest wall are still too tight, then I boost the dose of the SSRI. If the jaw and the psoas are still tight, then I boost the dose of the BuSpar. The BuSpar seems to affect muscles faster than the SSRI does. BuSpar dosages can be judged within two or three weeks, but SSRI adjustments take four to six weeks. I also adjust the dose of the nighttime medicine, such as BuSpar; this depends on how groggy the patient is in the morning and how they perceive their own sleep. It is interesting to observe how the different muscles react to the different classes and doses of medicines. Everyone is a little different; some people react to a minuscule dose, and some people need a regular or high dose.

Another condition sometimes associated with fibromyalgia is manic-depressive illness, or bipolar disorder. These patients often report "feeling strange" in reaction to even a partial dose of antidepressant. They don't like how they feel; they suffer a paradoxical reaction, that is, a side effect opposite from what is typical. In such cases I often use one of the new seizure drugs instead of an antidepressant. I have had pretty good results with Lamictal (lamotrigine), which is a seizure medicine that slightly increases one's energy. It helps with bipolar disorder by stabilizing the mood, and it also helps with fibromyalgia pain. Lamotrigine can result in a very rare but serious reaction called Stevens-Johnson syndrome, wherein the patient gets a bad rash and has to be hospitalized. This effect seems to depend on how quickly the dosage is increased. Increasing the dosage over a few months, up to 100 or 150 mg once a day, reduces the risk of the reaction to about one in ten thousand, which is acceptably low. Sometimes I add Topamax, another seizure drug, at a very low nighttime dose. Low-dose Topamax can help counteract the tendency to gain weight due to inactivity (a problem for women especially), and it also helps with disrupted sleep.

Many people with fibromyalgia become weather sensitive. We've discovered that low-dose Flexeril, low-dose Zanaflex (both muscle relaxants), or low-dose doxepin (an antidepressant) given at night seems to improve weather-induced stiffness. Many of my patients end up on that class of medicines from October until about May, when it's chilly and damp here in Seattle, or even during the summer if the weather warrants it. We use only about one-fourth of a 10-mg tablet of Flexeril—a really low dose. Zanaflex is typically indicated for MS-related spasticity, but it is now also used in chronic-headache or mixed-headache syndrome and in muscle-pain syndrome. Again, you don't need a large dose—about one-fourth or one-half of a 2-mg at night. The Zanaflex only lasts six hours, so if other drugs cause patients to feel groggy in the morning, then Zanaflex may be an option. However, it seems to be less effective than the others for treating weather sensitivity.

Some people, especially busy professionals, feel too sedated on a combination of an SSRI plus BuSpar plus a muscle relaxant. In such a case we may either switch the SSRI to Wellbutrin or add a low dose of Wellbutrin to the SSRI. It all depends upon how alert the patient must be during the day. About one-third of the population responds to Wellbutrin, but some people respond to SSRIs much better than they do to Wellbutrin, because the two classes work on different neurotransmitters. To figure out which works best for an individual, we try them on the SSRI, and if they have too many side effects, then we try the Wellbutrin. If their muscles get worse but they physically feel better, then we may reintroduce a low dose of the SSRI to the regimen once they've started with the Wellbutrin. Again, we use pretty low doses of most of these drugs; for example, I start the Wellbutrin at one-fourth of a 100-mg SR (slow release) in the morning. Most patients need only 100 or 150 mg in the morning, and none in the afternoon.

If after six to eight weeks the patient's muscles have relaxed a little bit, but they still experience prominent jaw problems, I might send them to biofeedback for three or four sessions to learn jaw relaxation. I also encourage them to try a little more physical activity. If traditional physical therapy aggravates their condition too much, I might refer them to an osteopath or a craniosacral practitioner to get them more active. Once they are doing better and walking more, then we try to improve their conditioning. Unless someone gets in shape and becomes almost an exercise fanatic, you can't really get them off the medicines. Exercise seems to double the effect of the antidepressant.

Sleep Aids

Interestingly, I can also tell from muscular tightness how well someone is sleeping. Sleep is important, but simply knocking a person out at night, while it may induce better sleep, doesn't improve their daytime functioning; they remain somewhat groggy. Some doctors believe that a solution to a lack of sleep is to thoroughly knock a patient out with Klonopin (traditionally an anti-seizure medication), but most patients I see who have been subjected to such a regimen are groggy. Sometimes they don't even realize how mentally slowed down they are until we get them off the long-acting stuff; then they realize, "Hey, I've been in a fog for the last year." I rarely use Klonopin for that reason; however, some people can tolerate it if they also suffer from an intense panic disorder or restless legs. So Klonopin can help, in a few cases. Additionally, Flexeril, Zanaflex, Celexa, and doxepin all help sleep.

It is pretty rare that I recommend Ativan as a sleeping medicine, but I do have a couple of patients on chronic Ativan and a few patients on chronic Ambien. I occasionally prescribe the antidepressant trazodone as a sleep aid, but it is not my favorite, because although it helps people sleep pretty well, it is ineffective as an antidepressant and as a muscle relaxant. However, it doesn't seem to cause much weight gain, which is a plus. Sometimes I use it along with an SSRI if the patient simply can't tolerate Flexeril or Zanaflex, but this is the case for only a minority of people. The same applies to Serzone. Some people do really well on Serzone, but because it's hard to find the right dose, it hasn't been my favorite.

All the SSRIs initially disrupt sleep, but once an individual has been on them for six or eight weeks, they actually sleep more deeply. This occurs because SSRIs help to regulate the whole serotonin metabolism and the primitive nervous system. The real action takes place in the primitive nervous system, because that is where people deal with stress.

Pain Medications

I prescribe pain medicines occasionally. However, if I have to rely on pain medicines, it means I haven't found the right combination of other drugs to normalize the myofascial textures and to allow people to exercise more, so usually pain medicines are a temporary measure. It usually takes three to four months for a patient relying on pain medication to feel better and function well.

Anti-inflammatories aren't very effective in treating fibromyalgia, and very few people are happy using only narcotics in the long term, because they tend to be depressants and can interfere with the thinking processes. Additionally, over the course of several months the effectiveness of narcotics seems to decrease. But they do play a role, and I do have a few people on chronic narcotics. I prescribe the whole spectrum of narcotics, from short-acting Vicodin to Oxycontin to methadone. The opiate Ultram is unusual in that it works better if the dosage is slowly built up and then maintained at a steady level, as opposed to using it "as needed," as you would a traditional pain pill. It affects some central-neurotransmitter modulators. Many of the seizure medicines also have pain-modulating qualities.

Natural Remedies

Some of my patients absolutely refuse to take prescription medicines, in which case they can go the naturopathic route. But at $150 to $200 per month with no insurance coverage, a regimen of natural supplements is expensive, and you don't know exactly what you're getting, since supplements aren't regulated. That's the drawback with the natural products.

In essence, these patients are doing the same sort of medical manipulations as we would with pharmaceuticals, except they're using such products as 5-HTP, supplemental magnesium, and amino acids. In some people, such a treatment can work quite well. I have seen patients who have done just as well on natural supplements as they did on prescription medicines.

Many FM patients might benefit from taking supplemental magnesium, malic acid, or a calcium-magnesium combination, as well as the B-complex vitamins and antioxidants. Dr. Andrew Weil's supplement plan seems reasonable, because it is true that a big segment of people with fibromyalgia are food sensitive. Wheat, other gluten-based products, and citrus are common allergens, so sometimes it is worth experimenting with eliminating those foods from one's diet.

FM in Men, Menopausal Women, and Young People

I believe that a lot of men have fibromyalgia. They complain about it differently—that is, there's a difference in how men report their symptoms—but if you actually look at their body and feel their muscle texture, you find fibromyalgia. The muscles of someone with FM typically have a "gritty," ropy, or fibrous texture; they feel like cooked meat. Skilled body workers can tell from the texture of the muscles whether an individual has fibromyalgia, regardless of the so-called tender points. Many areas not included in the classic tender points are abnormal in people with fibromyalgia. If you examine men on this basis, you will find that quite a few of them have fibromyalgia. They may call it back pain, headaches, or something else, but it is very similar. I have a number of male fibromyalgia patients. They respond well to medication manipulation along the lines of what I've discussed here.

Perimenopause and menopause create an interesting complication in women with FM. A hormonal correlation clearly exists in how people respond to dosages and manipulation of medication. Some perimenopausal and menopausal women who have been initially resistant to medicines will end up responding better to the same medicines after going on hormone replacement for a while.

I see surprisingly young patients with fibromyalgia. Many of these are the children of adult fibromyalgia patients; these youths show the telltale muscle changes as young as age thirteen or fourteen. A lot of young women who suffer from apparent disk disease in the neck turn out to be clenchers who have fibromyalgia. On average, FM patients present in their thirties, but the average age when the process that will ultimately be diagnosed as FM begins is probably in the late teenage years. If you can catch these kids early and teach them about biofeedback, posture, and exercises—teach them to take care of themselves—ideally they will end up better off than their parents did.

Conclusion

Although some doctors think of my program as "polypharmacy" (the use of multiple types of medicine to treat one condition) or as the placebo effect (because of the very low doses I prescribe), the bottom line for me is whether people function better after following my plan for a while. Approximately 70 percent of my fibromyalgia patients have gotten better.

The main thing patients tell me about how my treatment plan has helped them is that they are able to do more without paying for it a day or two later with severe pain that requires bed rest. They tell me, "Now I can hike five miles and carry a backpack, or I can do gardening and not pay for it later." Basically, I know how they are doing by the amount of aerobic activity they can tolerate. And that's how I judge success—by the kind of life my patients are living.

▲▲▲

TAKING PART IN A STUDY

Taking part in valid clinical research gives chronically ill patients an opportunity to contribute to the advancement of medical science. And as the experience of Diane H. shows (below), participants in a clinical trial involving a potential new treatment may also gain some relief from their symptoms, if the treatment proves beneficial.

If you consider participating in a clinical trial, take care to get detailed information about the procedures involved and about your rights and responsibilities as a participant. You will most likely be asked to attend a screening interview. Make a list of questions to take with you. These might include:

◀ What is the purpose of the study?

◀ Who is sponsoring the study?

◀ What are the benefits and risks of the treatment being researched? What are the possible side effects?

◀ How much time will be required of me per week/month?

◀ Exactly what procedures will be involved?

◀ Will any of the procedures be painful?

◀ Will my participation require any hospital stays?

◀ Do I continue taking my current medications and/or supplements?

◀ Will I incur any expenses for participating? Will I be paid for participating?

Some of these issues will likely be addressed in the literature given to you by the researchers. One item they will give you is called an *informed-consent document*, which essentially details the procedures involved, tells how long the trial will last, and outlines the risks and benefits expected from the treatment. The researchers will also screen you for eligibility. Your symptoms, age, medical history, etc., may or may not meet the exact criteria they're looking for.

I have participated in several studies through the University of Washington. One was part of a sleep-dysfunction study funded by the National Institute of Nursing Research. The study examined growth hormone and prolactin, two hormones, as mentioned in Chapter 4, that are often found in lower-than-normal amounts in FM patients. As a subject, I had to keep a month-long journal of my sleep habits and symptoms. Once I qualified, I had to go off all of my medications so the researchers could get a good idea of my hormone levels without any interference. That was the difficult part! I didn't mind sleeping in the lab with all of the electrodes stuck into my skin and on my head.

I also took part in a study of couples examining how CFS affects both partners in the ways we take care of household and daily tasks. Since a chronic illness affects both the patient and her or his partner, participating in this study seemed appropriate and timely.

Diane H. recently participated in a six-month study sponsored by the University of Arizona College of Medicine. It focused on homeopathy and its effects on FM. Here are a few of her comments, written while the study was still going on:

Diane H.   I will soon be finished with my participation in this double-blind, placebo-controlled study. I am feeling so good, and I'm very excited about this treatment. Upon first starting the homeopathic formula being researched, however, I endured the "month from hell." All my symptoms flared up, but then they slowly settled down, and four weeks later I was feeling great again. Then came four more hellish days of insomnia, aching, and fatigue, and then I started to feel good once again.

The doctors explained that the remedy works in "waves"—that there will be ups and downs for a while, and then the number of good days increases and the number of bad days decreases. For me, a good day consists of falling asleep easily, sleeping through the night, waking up feeling rested instead of fatigued, having the energy to walk and exercise, an absence of heartburn, achiness but no pain, and clear cognitive functioning. I can think, focus, prioritize, organize, concentrate, and remember something for more than thirty seconds. I haven't felt this good mentally in years.

The doctor warned that although I was feeling better, it would take years for my immune system to "repair," and that I still need to slow down, pace myself, take care of myself, and minimize my stress levels as best I can.

▲▲▲

ONGOING RESEARCH

It is encouraging to realize that potential new treatments for fibromyalgia are always being studied. In this section and the next one, two FM experts—one the CEO of a health-products company and the other an assistant professor at a major teaching hospital—describe some of the latest clinical research.

Dennis Schoen is CEO of Pro Health, Inc., which publishes the newsletter *Healthwatch* and sponsors the excellent website www.ImmuneSupport.com. The company also funds and raises money for FM and CFS research and community support. Pro Health has grown into the largest retailer of specialty FM- and CFS-focused products, including dietary supplements, the Alpha Stim microcurrent unit, the Cuddle Ewe line of wool-batting bed accessories, and other health products (see Resources).

Here, Schoen reports on some of the latest studies he's aware of involving treatment options for fibromyalgia:

▲▲▲

I am fortunate to be able to attend the important fibromyalgia and chronic fatigue syndrome research conferences and to interact with top researchers in conventional and alternative medicine, as well as with pharmaceutical executives. The most pervasive trend I see in both FM and CFS research is the focus on understanding the causes of the diseases as well as the development of some exciting treatment options. I understand that one of the pharmaceutical giants is working on a fibromyalgia-specific drug that might be approved for release in 2003. Another pharmaceutical company, Cypress BioScience, Inc., has dedicated its product-research efforts entirely to fibromyalgia.

A very interesting clinical study is under way of a procedure that might provide relief for sudden-onset FM, although the results may be unavailable for another year or so. Many patients appear to benefit from the Flexyx Neurotherapy System (FNS). FNS is both a brain-wave biofeedback system and a treatment system. It has been in use for over a decade, but these will be the first clinical results on its effectiveness. FNS is for patients with central nervous system (CNS) dysfunction who suffer pain as well as impairments to their cognitive functioning, mood, energy, movement (paralysis), and balance. As a treatment system it measures brain waves and directs the waves to send back to the patient a reflection of those waves. The data is transmitted via a very weak FM-radio signal, so there's nothing to watch or feel. FNS makes use of the natural, unconscious self-regulation patterns already present in our brain and nervous system and resets them so that they can once again work well. There's nothing the person receiving FNS needs to do. The brain already knows how to do it, and it just needs a little nudge to work well again.

Brain waves are generated by the subcortex (the inner portions of the brain) in response to physical trauma or viruses. When trauma such as a head injury occurs, the brain tries to defend itself against the brain waves caused by the trauma by throwing up neurochemical barriers in the cortex (the outer surfaces of the brain). As we age, these neurochemicals lose their effectiveness. With a weakened defense, the cortex becomes overwhelmed by these brain waves, and the brain starts to misinterpret signals from the body.

In an FM patient, ordinary signals resulting from physical stimuli are interpreted as pain. The problem is how the brain manages and identifies stimulation. The brain's map of the body becomes scrambled and confused when the cortex is overwhelmed by brain waves. What the FNS does is to stimulate the cortex with reflected brain waves, helping to correct the confusion, making it clear that the signal the cortex received was not a pain signal. The brain then begins to recognize the differences and to correct the confused signals itself.

FNS stimulates the cortex so that it regains competence, as well as a sense of how to react to stimuli. In addition, the origin of pain patterns gets a more accurate representation. Then the cortex resumes its primary job of inhibiting subcortical activities. The FNS does not correct physical abnormalities; it teaches the cortex to compensate for a whole host of problems.

Once the brain starts to function normally, two things happen. First, the brain correctly identifies the signals it gets from the body, as well as the sources of those signals. So the brain becomes able to tell the difference between an ordinary muscle signal and a pain signal, and it stops sensing pain where there are just ordinary sensations. For example, it stops equating, say, an ordinary shoulder sensation with a pain in the jaw. Second, because the brain and nervous system are no longer barraged by false pain and confusion signals, they become relieved of the jobs of trying to sort through all the confused signals and of controlling signals that don't need to be controlled. This makes living immensely easier by lowering the workload of the brain and nervous system. When living and ordinary tasks become easier and get done faster, people have more energy and feel less irritable, angry, frustrated, and depressed.

Another very interesting fibromyalgia treatment is undergoing clinical trials at the University of Minnesota. A physician who treats many patients suffering from chronic pain noticed that his female fibromyalgia patients who became pregnant reported remission of their symptoms when they were pregnant and the return of their symptoms within one or two months after delivery. After seeing this trend repeated over the years, the physician began to search for any agent or hormone within the body that would have an effect on the collagen of connective tissues. In doing so he became acquainted with a little-known pregnancy hormone called relaxin, which in most mammals is produced in ten times greater quantity during pregnancy. Its main purpose is to facilitate birth by relaxing the pelvic ligaments. The hormone is now marketed as the supplement Vitalaxin. Results from the study of this product for treating FM are due in late 2002.

Other studies have been completed or are under way on products to assist FM patients:

◄ Jon Russell, M.D., recently completed a study on the Cuddle Ewe line of bedding accessories. (Pro Health is a retailer of Cuddle Ewe products.) In his conclusion he wrote, "[T]here was significant increase in sleep quality and quantity with the Cuddle Ewe device."

◄ A non-antigen-specific transfer factor product known as transfer factor basics is being studied to determine if it can raise natural killer–cell function. Since nearly 70 percent of FM patients have CFS symptoms, maintaining overall immune health is key to supporting the body's fragile immune system.

A LOOK AT MORE FM STUDIES

Kim Dupree-Jones, R.N., Ph.D., F.N.P., is an assistant professor at the Oregon Health & Science University School of Nursing in Portland. She tells us about some of the current studies concerning FM treatment possibilities that she's involved in:

Growth-Hormone Studies

One of our current studies looks at the brain's failure to release its natural stores of growth hormone either during a pharmacologic challenge or during an exercise challenge. Failure to release growth hormones has implications for the symptoms that go with fibromyalgia. For example, growth hormones are known to have the effect of building bigger, stronger muscles. But fibromyalgia patients apparently fail to produce the beautiful surge of growth hormone that is normal in response to a pharmacologic challenge, the stress of exercise, or at night during deep sleep. So FM patients are set up hormonally to experience less restorative sleep, muscle pain, and soreness, including delayed-onset muscle soreness, and all the general fatigue and bad feeling that goes with having inadequate release of growth hormone. One of our preliminary studies looked at actually supplementing fibromyalgia patients with injectable growth hormone. A number of women with fibromyalgia received either injectable growth hormone or an injectable placebo. After nine months, we saw that the people who got the growth hormone, as opposed to the placebo, had a much better response to pain measures and other system measures. In other words, they felt a lot better.

The problem with that study was threefold. The first was that growth-hormone supplementation costs almost a thousand dollars per month, and insurance won't touch it. Second, it has to be given by injection, and although giving oneself shots every day is doable, it's less than ideal. Third, a very small number of people who take growth hormones endure the side effect of fluid retention. This is particularly a problem for patients who suffer chronic pain and are prone to complications such as carpal-tunnel syndrome, because fluid retention can worsen carpal-tunnel syndrome. Because of these three drawbacks, we wanted to look for another medication or another marker which might show the same positive results as injectable growth hormone yet be more cost effective and cause fewer side effects.

We went to the literature on growth-hormone deficiency and saw that it is often diagnosed with a medication called Mestinon (pyridostigmine bromide), which is most commonly given for the treatment of myasthenia gravis. In the FM population, it works centrally at the hypothalamus by decreasing another hormone called somatostatin. Increased somatostatin levels keep growth hormones from being released. When we can pharmacologically alter the levels of somatostatin, then people with fibromyalgia can release their own growth hormone instead of taking an expensive injectable treatment. In the first study we did, FM patients were given a low dose of Mestinon. It basically normalized their growth-hormone response to exercise. We then decreased the dose even further, again with favorable results. What's important about that study is that it indicates more firmly that fibromyalgia is a problem of the brain and the spinal cord; it's a problem of the central nervous system rather than a problem of the muscles and the peripheral nervous system. There is no question that peripheral muscle pain exists and that it is a major problem in FM, but it is probably not the origin of the muscle problem. The origin is probably in the brain and spinal cord. Basically the medication made the people with fibromyalgia look like the people without fibromyalgia; in other words, it normalized their growth-hormone response. So that was very exciting to us.

Modifying Exercise for the FM Patient

We have done exercise studies and have learned that there is a very specific way in which women with fibromyalgia need to exercise to avoid an increase in delayed-onset muscle soreness. One reason people with fibromyalgia have so much trouble exercising is that most exercise is geared to the general population. It's too intense, too high impact, and involves movements that occur too far away from the midline of the body—that is, it involves an excess of eccentric muscle work, which causes muscle microtrauma. Eccentric muscle contraction is the phase in which the muscle is contracted while it is elongated, such as when walking down a steep hill or having the arms above the head to pull down a weight or reach a high surface. We've designed three exercise programs for people with fibromyalgia: one for stretching, one for strength training, and one for aerobics. Our programs keep the intensity low and keep the movements near the midline of the body to decrease the amount of eccentric work. All three were developed by Dr. Sharon Clark, who is an exercise physiologist with years of experience in fibromyalgia research. Instructional videotapes for each of the programs are available through the website of the Oregon Fibromyalgia Foundation (OFF), www.myalgia.com. Dr. Robert Bennett, a founding member of the OFF, provides an introduction and conclusion on the videos. He represented Oregon Health & Science University in a multisite study that developed the American College of Rheumatology 1990 diagnostic criteria for FM. One of our current grants will let us conduct a placebo-controlled study of our exercise program plus a regimen of pyridostigmine bromide (Mestinon) to see if treatment involving both remedies is more effective than either one in isolation.

Studying Chronic Pain

My colleagues and I are currently working on a study called "Pain Similarities in Breast Cancer and Fibromyalgia." Women survive breast cancer now longer than they ever have. The five-year survival rate presently surpasses 90 percent for noninvasive cancer, and because women with breast cancer are living longer after initial diagnosis and treatment, quality of life is very important, specifically in regards to chronic pain after breast cancer surgery. We want to know if such postsurgery pain is a local or a regional issue related to nerve damage from surgery, or if "crossover" occurs in the brain so that what used to be regional pain now turns into widespread pain. We're using a machine called a dermal sensory analyzer that looks at sensations of hot and cold and vibration in the nerve receptors at skin level to tell us when the transfer from regional to widespread pain occurs. The study will help us pilot test the machine and will give us more information about the characteristics and history of women with fibromyalgia after breast cancer surgery versus those who suffer only regional pain after breast cancer surgery. With this, we hope to better understand and develop diagnostic assessments of women following breast cancer surgery to figure out who is at high risk for developing fibromyalgia and to treat them more aggressively for postsurgery chronic pain.

In trying out new treatments for ailments such as fibromyalgia, it's not good enough to just say, "Here's our theory; we know it works, so we use it in our clinical practice." Medical and science professionals really need to obtain the backing to do randomized control trials; that is how science is advanced.

Websites for FM'ers

If readers want to ask me questions about managing their illness, they can visit the website www.WebMD.com; then click on "message boards," and then on "Fibromyalgia/Chronic Fatigue: Dr. Kim Jones." There they can see posts from about three thousand other FM patients from all over the world and my responses to their questions about medication, therapy, exercise, etc. This message board is so powerful because the advice is not from doctor or nurse to patient. It's from people who have figured out the tricks of living well with fibromyalgia. I might suggest a certain medication, for example, and then someone who actually has the illness will post and say, "Yeah, Kim is right, but the thing that really helps me more is to use a cup with a certain sort of lid, because my hands are really shaky." I don't want to downplay my role on the message board, but it also features people helping other people, and I think visitors sometimes get more out of that than from medical advice.

I'm also involved in another website, www.fibromyalgia.com. We want to be a clearinghouse for fibromyalgia information. If a health-care provider finished school more than about five years ago, there is a good chance they received no instruction about fibromyalgia whatsoever, and an even greater chance that they lack awareness of the latest research on central sensitization and on how the brain and spinal cord are affected electrically, chemically, and hormonally in people who have chronic, widespread pain. The majority of health-care providers in the community probably feel pretty helpless about how to take care of their patients with FM. Fortunately, some treatments now exist that are working, and we want to get the word out.

Dr. Jones also offers these thoughts on a scientifically sound hypothesis regarding a potential therapy versus anecdotal evidence or testimonial:

▲▲▲

Testimonials about treatments are fine, and what makes them stronger is to be able to say whether the treatment in question is or is not supported by the medical literature. The OFF website (www.myalgia.com) includes many such examples—for instance, is it worth your time and money to buy blue-green algae? Is it worth your time and money to buy this herb or that vitamin? Has it really been tested? Robert Bennett does a good job of putting very scientific, could-be-confusing information into language for the layperson. Patients get so frustrated when they spend hundreds of dollars on a pain cream or some other remedy they've seen advertised on a TV infomercial and it doesn't work. The people we see are often on disability; they are underemployed for their education because chronic pain has taken such a toll, so we are on a personal crusade to help people make scientifically sound decisions regarding their treatments.

▲▲▲

A NATUROPATHIC APPROACH: TREATMENT WITH ENZYMES

Naturopathic medicine (also called naturopathy) emphasizes the inherent healing capacity of the patient. The word *naturopathy* was first used in the United States about a hundred years ago, but the therapies used by naturopathic physicians and the underlying philosophies of naturopathy are ancient. The concept of "nature as healer"—a central tenet of naturopathy—forms the basis of the medicine practiced by many indigenous cultures around the world. Naturopathic doctors historically have used herbs, food, water, fasting, and tissue manipulation to treat their patients. Modern practitioners continue to use these therapies as their primary tools and in addition conduct and make use of the latest biochemical research involving nutrition, botanicals, and other natural treatments. With the creation by the U.S. Congress of the Office of Alternative Medicine in 1992, naturopathy and other complementary therapies are enjoying "official" recognition of their effectiveness and widespread popularity.

Dr. Jenefer Scripps Huntoon is a naturopathic physician who graduated from the National College of Naturopathy in 1975 and practices in Seattle. She specializes in the treatment of digestive problems, gastrointestinal disorders, autoimmune conditions, and fibromyalgia. She has developed a program of supplementation with enzymes, which she discusses below, along with her recommendations for diet.

My colleagues and I, who are certified as plant-enzyme specialists, use supplementary plant enzymes in two specific ways. The first is as an aid to proper digestion, and the second is to accomplish a therapeutic purpose, such as cleaning up the undigested protein and carbohydrate in the blood, or binding with toxins to pull them out.

Digestive enzymes are necessary for the digestion of fat, carbohydrates, protein, and fiber. Undigested food creates particles that act like poisons in the body. This can cause inflammation and musculoskeletal pain. Enzymes are also important for absorption of micronutrients, that is, vitamins and minerals. People who are deficient in certain nutrients are susceptible to musculoskeletal pain such as that associated with fibromyalgia. For example, enzymes are necessary for proper digestion of vitamin C. If a person is low in vitamin C, her or his joints become weak, because vitamin C is needed to strengthen connective tissue. A person deficient in vitamin C also is more prone to viruses. For this reason, in addition to using enzymes, we also use vitamins therapeutically to help reduce inflammation.

We use an enzyme formula that's high in amylase—which aids in the digestion of carbohydrate, which in turn helps joint flexibility—and high in protease, which aids in the digestion of protein. Undigested protein in the blood leads to high levels of uric acid, a condition that feels like having fiberglass in the blood, causing joint pain. Proper digestion of protein, on the other hand, helps reduce inflammation. Another important function of protein is its role in making immunoglobulins, which support the immune system. Protein is also used to make hormones. Individuals who fail to digest proteins properly often suffer from a suppressed immune system and from hormonal imbalances. We also use the enzyme cellulase to bind with toxins and pull them out of the tissues—not toxins from undigested food, but rather lead, mercury, cadmium, aluminum, preservatives, and the like.

As you can see, proper digestion of all the components of food—carbohydrate, fat, protein, vitamins, and minerals—is very important in an overall treatment plan for fibromyalgia symptoms such as inflammation, musculoskeletal pain and stiffness, and suppressed immune functioning.

I don't necessarily regard all fibromyalgia patients as requiring the same treatment. I've had some patients who felt better after two days of treatment, and some patients who took a month or two to experience a change. Typically, FM patients will feel better after about two weeks on my program, but there are many variables in individuals' physiology. I did a structural alignment on a fibromyalgia patient who felt better the next day. She came to me for structural alignment about six weeks in a row, and she took the enzymes I recommended, and she's feeling better than ever. She is able to go back to work and to do all kinds of things she couldn't before. I think she had more of a spinal problem than an enzyme problem or a nutritional problem. In some FM cases, it's a combination of things.

Diet is important—for FM patients and everyone else. I can put a patient on all the right remedies, and they may feel somewhat better, but working with diet is really important to effect a substantial change in a person's health. In general I recommend eating natural, whole foods instead of white flour and processed foods; in other words, if you are going to eat rice, select brown rice over white rice. If you eat bread, eat whole-grain bread instead of white bread.

Most people need to reduce the amount of sugar in their diet, which is a challenge because sugar is so addictive. But the better a patient is able to comply with a more nutritious diet and to eliminate sugar, the better everything else will work. Sugar depletes the body because it offers no nutritive value, it lowers the immune system, and it causes candida yeast that leads to muscle and joint pain. Sugar wreaks havoc by allowing candida yeast to grow out of control. Candida yeast occurs in the body normally, but if it is fed, it takes over and becomes a problem, causing a lowered immune system and musculoskeletal pain. A lot of people don't realize that the sugar in fruit juice is almost as bad as table sugar. Too much fruit sugar also feeds candida yeast. People need to limit fruit to perhaps two servings a day and to load up on vegetables. As a replacement for sugar we recommend stevia, which is an herbal sweetener. It tastes sweet, can be taken by diabetics, and helps a person lose the craving for sweets. It seems to help get people off sugar. It's a crutch they can use that's safe.

Pharmaceutical and herbal treatments can be used to kill candida yeast, but these remedies by themselves don't necessarily solve the problem. I have seen people on nystatin, a typical drug used to get rid of yeast. The drug kills the yeast, but the yeast can come back as an even stronger strain if the patient doesn't also change his or her diet. Diet is extremely crucial in treating candida, but if patients can tolerate them, there are a number of herbs, botanicals, and enzymes that will speed up the process of getting the yeast under control.

We have our own specific plant-enzyme remedies that are very effective in counteracting yeast. In particular, we use protease—the protein-digesting enzyme—but it's a powerful formula and cannot be taken by people with a sensitive stomach. It's unavailable over the counter. However, all kinds of anticandida formulas are available over the counter in health stores, including oil of oregano and tea-tree oil.

In conclusion, much chronic degenerative disease is a result of a diet high in cooked and processed foods. The key to maintaining optimal health is to eat fruit, vegetables, nuts, and seeds in the raw, unprocessed state whenever possible. Since it is difficult in our society to eat a diet of the recommended 75 percent raw foods, it helps to supplement with a plant-enzyme formula. Plant enzymes predigest food, reduce the need for the body to produce hydrochloric acid and pancreatic enzymes, prevent chronic degenerative disease, and slow the aging process. We have been able to greatly reduce the number of vitamin and mineral tablets people need by supplementing with plant enzymes, which complete the assimilation of the nutritional tablets as well as the proper assimilation of food. In digestion and energy metabolism, enzymes truly are the missing link.

(A portion of the information contained in this essay was excerpted from an article by Dr. Huntoon that appeared in Well-Being Journal, *volume II, number 1, March/April 1993.)*

ENERGY THERAPY

Western health practitioners are placing ever more emphasis on treating the whole person: body, mind, emotions, and spirit. An exciting new development in the holistic approach to health is energy therapy, which combines Western modes of psychotherapy with the Eastern method of correcting a patient's life-force energy, the same energy system that forms the basis of the ancient Chinese healing techniques of acupuncture and acupressure.

Marti MacEwan, M.A., L.M.H.C., is a Licensed Mental Health Counselor who has been in private practice in Seattle for over twenty years. She gives us this overview of energy therapy:

▲▲▲

Energy therapy is a new method of psychotherapy based on the growing field of energy psychology. In the majority of cases, energy therapy dramatically reduces specific emotional distress and restores emotional well-being by clearing disturbances in the body's electromagnetic energy systems. In a nutshell: When your body's energy is balanced and clear, your emotional distress diminishes and you feel better. Then you can approach your life with more emotional well-being and mental clarity. In recent years, I have studied energy therapy with leaders in the field, mastering their techniques and developing variations of my own. I have found that adding energy therapy to traditional "talk" therapy has been extremely effective.

Energy therapy can be quite helpful in bringing relief to a person suffering from a chronic illness such as fibromyalgia. When someone has a chronic disease—especially a chronic disease that directly affects the amount of energy the person has—resolving painful mental-health issues is very important for overall healing.

Your mental and emotional health, of course, cannot be separated from your physical health, since one affects the other in many profound and complex ways. Naturally, when your life changes dramatically with the onset of a chronic illness and you become subject to many physical limitations you didn't have before, you are likely to experience painful emotions about it: upset, loss, sadness, disappointment, resentment, anger, fear, depression. In that way, your physical condition directly affects your mental health.

In turn, your mental health affects your physical condition. Experiencing uncomfortable, draining, negative emotions and thinking uncomfortable, draining, negative thoughts simply adds to the weight of your already burdensome condition. The stress of negative thoughts and emotions takes a toll on the body and can make the condition worse. They drain your energy—which is exactly what you need to preserve. You need every bit of energy for living your daily life with all its usual issues, and, most importantly, you need that energy for healing.

So your painful emotions on the one hand and your painful physical condition on the other can continually affect each other and keep you from moving forward in your healing process. Something has to break this cycle. That's where energy therapy comes in.

It is commonly accepted by many health practitioners that each of us has a powerful and complex energy system that permeates and radiates from our bodies—the same flow of energy that is utilized and treated in acupuncture and acupressure. This energy system is invisible to us (at least to most of us), but many believe that it is concretely and demonstrably real. The condition of our energy system affects us immediately and profoundly. It has everything to do with how we feel. When the flow of our energy system is balanced and clear, we feel good, we "hum," our energy is strong, and we have plenty of personal power.

Negative thoughts and emotions can remain lodged in the energy system. Whether they come from past traumatic experiences, patterns of emotional response from childhood, present-day circumstances, or our reactions to the disease itself, they take energy for us to deal with. You can think of it as energy that is tied up and therefore unavailable for present-day healing. It is also negative energy that is blocking the positive thoughts and feelings that have been shown to have concrete healing effects. So, the more a person with a chronic illness can resolve her negativity—however justified it is given the changes in her life—the more energy is available to her for feeling her best and, just possibly, for healing from her disease.

What energy therapy does, in the words of one of my clients, is to "evaporate" the old emotional wounds and negative beliefs of the past. When energy therapy works its best, you are able to truly say of your emotional pain, "That was then; this is now." You are able to get to what I call a "new normal," where recurrent, debilitating, painful emotions simply no longer affect you, and you no longer experience their draining influence. Energy that once was used to maintain and struggle with those negative feelings has

been "freed" and is now available for use in your present-day healing. When we add this element to the traditional counseling or
therapy process, recovery is more rapid, pain-free, and complete
than we have ever experienced before.

Energy therapy, as I practice it, is a combination of traditional
counseling and energy-clearing methods. This blend allows you to
talk about, understand, and honor your emotional distress, as in
traditional therapy, and then to gently release your painful feelings
from where they are lodged in your energy system, so you are no
longer under the influence of your limiting emotions. You are then
free to truly recover; you can feel better, act, and react the way you
intend to, and make healthier, more positive choices. When your
energy is clear and there is no disturbance in your energy field, in
the presence of a thought, memory, or emotion, you feel completely different from how you're used to feeling. For example:

◀ You are able to think (more) clearly.

◀ You can see options and possibilities you couldn't see
before.

◀ You are able to take action.

◀ You have no more emotional distress about the issue.

I combine a number of approaches in the energy part of my
work. These include Thought Field Therapy, an acupuncture
meridian–based method without the needles; Energy Medicine,
which corrects and balances the auric field, chakra system, and
other energies in the body; and Shifting the Assemblage Point,
which reorients the entire energy field around the heart center,
subtly but powerfully initiating an overall healing process. When
I use these specific and painless techniques to correct and balance
a client's energy system while she is focusing on an issue or problem, she can very often actually feel the uncomfortable emotions
subside.

If you are interested in exploring more about each of these
approaches, please visit my website at www.energytherapist.com.

The site includes information, book recommendations, and links to other websites, including referral sites, where you can find the name and phone number of an energy therapist in your region.

▲▲▲

Energy psychology is a growing field, so you should be able to find a practitioner in your area. Check out the links on Marti Mac-Ewan's website. Additionally, an acupuncturist, chiropractor, or massage therapist who is aware of alternative-health techniques may be able to give you more information.

I hope this chapter has encouraged you to continue your search for FM treatment breakthroughs. Consider informing yourself about fibromyalgia news on a regular basis by subscribing to a reputable newsletter or two (see Resources). Keeping abreast of the latest developments in FM research and treatment is one way to stay proactive in our self-care.

Life Goes On

I am especially lucky to have my cousin Linda in my life. It was a shock to find out that she, too, had FM. We were diagnosed the same year. Linda also battles bipolar disorder and chronic fatigue syndrome, and she tells me that she will not let her illnesses get in the way of living a full life. "I am a strong person and I deserve to be healthy and happy," she says. "I did not cause my FM, but I *can* take good care of myself. FM has taught me to slow down."

Like Linda, I believe I have FM for a reason. When I look back over my life (and I have been doing this a lot lately since I'm creeping up on age forty), I try to think of the last ten years as a quarter of my life spent learning how to live in a balanced and healthier way. I am determined to find a positive in my situation; doing so helps me to feel like I have some control over the pain.

BEYOND FIBROMYALGIA

When I think about my life beyond living with fibromyalgia, I focus on the positive things I have learned. To focus on anything else would be less than constructive, and my goal is to get better while learning about myself along the way. I also focus on what makes me happy: A walk at night with my dogs. Thoughts of the beach cabins we visit each year. One-upping my antiques-collecting friends by comparing who got the oldest, cheapest, coolest junk over the weekend. Watching my tabby cats. Rhyming really bad songs and poems for my pets and friends. E-mailing with my FM friends. As soon as I stopped fighting against having FM and understood that I might as well get on with the business of living, my life changed.

Gerry L. I really have to think about what I do for myself beyond treating FM. Fighting the illness has taken so much of my time. It is all consuming. At times I can see or think of nothing else. I have said that I have FM, but FM is not me. It is hard to make that distinction. Some of the things I have done to help me manage FM— for example, drumming, tai chi, meditation, guided relaxation, etc.—I would do even if I did not have FM. They have become part of me and I enjoy them. Yet I still am searching for more purpose and meaning in my life.

Cydney B. I was able to be a caregiver to my father-in-law, which would not have happened if I had been working. We would have hired someone.

I was able to explore my lifelong desire to write, and I would still like to do so, but my energy wanes a little more each year.

I was able to be near my daughter when she had a miscarriage and got divorced, which I would not have been able to do if I had been working.

I was able to help my brother when he was battling cancer. I can come to the aid of any family member (who doesn't require a lot of physical care) without hesitation or worrying about work.

I am a different person from who I would have been had I stayed on my other path. I think I like this person better—other than the physical weakness.

Patricia S. The only thing positive I can say about illness is that it teaches you how important health is. Someone who is pain-free and in good health takes it for granted. I don't think there is a way to teach that to anyone. It's something you learn from experience. I've learned that you have to live with the illness because there is no alternative except death, which is not something I'm ready for. You go on with life, and you're more accepting of what you've been dealt. I have learned what a good guy my boyfriend is to have stuck with me through this, even though it's been tough. But I do not feel that being ill has made me a better person.

Sisu G. Jack Benny gave a speech in which he said, "I don't deserve this award. But then, I don't deserve arthritis, and I've got that, too." I still don't know how to fit the concept of a chronic illness into my worldview. It threw me for a loop—I don't deserve this. Nobody deserves this; how can it happen? And maybe it's not about deserving. If bad things happened only to bad people, no one would have any cause for compassion.

Even if this FM lasts my whole expected life span, my quality of life will continue to improve as I get a better handle on how to adapt and how to accommodate my new limits.

Victoria M. I am more accepting of less perfection. I look for the simple pleasures these days. I have more appreciation of what I can achieve rather than chasing what I cannot.

Sonia H. For several years, I was scared, angry, and resentful. Now I feel acceptance for the most part, but disappointment about what might have been.

Diane H. I'm no longer mad, although I was initially angry at the loss of my energy and cognitive functioning. I now see FM as a blessing. It has led me to a more peaceful, less stressful existence, inside and out. I'm not scared, because FM is not degenerative and not life-threatening. I don't feel alone. I have a loving, supportive husband and three sisters with FM as a support group. I don't resent my illness or anyone or anything. If anything, FM has taught me self-acceptance and patience with myself.

▲▲▲

WHAT KEEPS US GOING?

I don't spent much time thinking about the possibility of a cure for fibromyalgia. My reality is right here in my body. However, once in a while, I do permit myself to dream about it. When that day comes, I'm sure I will see the headlines blaring across magazine covers. Until then, I keep taking my medications, doing my exercises, and staying positive.

My partner says I was excited when I announced I could walk a block. I don't remember that night. Just like I can't remember what it's like not to have pain in my feet. If you have FM, you know just what I mean. It sounds unthinkable, but you get used to having the pain with you, all day, every day. In the face of that knowledge, what keeps me going is an unshakable knowledge that I will achieve a good remission. I have seen it happen; it's not an urban legend! A person's symptoms check out, one at a time. Soon after my diagnosis, a member of my support group told us she woke up one morning knowing something was different, and then she realized that her pain was gone. She enjoyed a fairly long remission; it happened after she completely changed her life.

And what keeps me going is the knowledge that I have adjusted my life to a point where even if this is the best I'm going to get, health-wise, I am okay with it for now. I have to be. What is the alternative? As long as I work at getting better by exercising, taking my medications and supplements, watching my diet, and working on my mental health, I know that I am on the right track.

Sisu G. It's unrealistic to expect that I will have this illness for the rest of my life. Medical knowledge is growing exponentially. It's reasonable to expect a cure in the next ten to fifteen years. In the meantime, I guess my hopes have toned down a bit. Still, I feel good about the future. I work enough things around the edges to feel like I'm leading a productive life. Hell, I went out and got houseplants. I'm home to water them on Friday nights.

It's really difficult to dream big when I can't do the laundry. But I try to at least dream. I try to think that there will be more to my life than this. It's not about surviving; it's about still being able to laugh. When I grow up, I want to be outrageous. I want to be a cheerful old lady, the annoying kind who makes you laugh in the post-office line because she says something completely out of order to the clerk. When I grow up, I want to be a rock star. A novelist. A grandma who embarrasses her relatives by dressing in low-cut, high-heeled streaks of wild abandon. I want to be in the way. I want to be exactly who I am now, only more so. And I want to somehow get my life back between now and then so that I can do all this. I practice a little at a time. I figure I'd better have it down by then, because I certainly won't waste any of my newfound energy on practicing!

Gerry L. What drives me to go forward every day? Me! It's my turn! My natural instinct, because I am a survivor. Sometimes I wind up in neutral, and other times it feels like reverse, but I shift right back into forward! Life itself keeps me going. Just look around; look up to the sky and look down to Mother Earth. Take it all in. The universe is full of wonders. Wow! What is it all about? What is the essence of this natural scene—not just the plants and animals, but the whole of it all?

Life is there whether I have FM or not. So why let it pass me by? You may think this is simplifying it, and one's outlook does depend on the severity of symptoms and pain level on any given day. Mine does. I'm still up and down. The struggle is still there. But I don't want to miss out.

Jean T. I get up each morning looking forward to the day. Since I don't have the pain I have had in the past, it is easier to be optimistic. My family is very important to me. I look forward to seeing my grandsons and my great-grandchildren.

Cydney B. Quite frankly, with my family history, waking up alive every morning is a pretty good reward. I recently turned fifty-four. My mother died at fifty-three, my father at forty-six. My older brother and sister and I were always a little doubtful we'd outlive our parents, and now that all three of us have done so, it feels great. I love birthdays! They're better than the alternative.

I am driven by a need to get to my deathbed at a ripe old age and say, "Well, that was fun." I want to make this life as much fun as I can. And I want to also get to the end and have people say, "She was a good person." You can still do those things, even if you're sick.

Charlene M. I try to do things that I love. I try to enjoy simple things, like sitting in my swing in the backyard and enjoying the weather, summer or winter.

I think my kids are my main reason for going on. I don't want to be a burden to them, but I also want to be able to enjoy them. The small things have become more important to me, such as seeing my grandchildren's smiling faces. My heart just jerks every time they are glad to see me.

Val T. I have learned to pamper myself when needed. What drives me forward every day is fear of giving in. I feel I would be a failure if I gave up. I will continue to fight for the rest of my life! The alternative would be to stay home, and that would destroy me mentally and physically.

Victoria M. The love I have for my children is what drives me forward every day. I have to set an example. They are young and must learn how to overcome life's obstacles constructively and appropriately. Sharing my children's joys and achievements, watching them grow and develop into such remarkable human beings is my greatest reward. All my hard work is reflected in my children.

To a lesser extent, but nonetheless an important catalyst for me, is the need for change in our society. I feel a huge desire and need to inform and support others, to help change the face of medicine and advocate for the rights of the chronically ill.

Beyond treating my FM, I am planning my future as a well person. I am quite determined to overcome this condition and to find the causes, to educate and support others, and to establish a clinic for chronically ill people. I want to make a difference. Not everyone is as "stubborn" or as able as I have been, and I believe we should use life's experiences to learn and to work to make our society more loving, accepting, and supportive.

Emma L. I do nothing special for myself other than eating as much chocolate as I want and being close to nature as often as I can. I think that just taking care of my basic everyday needs under very adverse circumstances is already doing a lot for myself, and waking up every day still here makes me live another day as best I can. Not having gone to the nuthouse is my main reward.

Lalenya R. What drives me forward is my family, as well as the hope that researchers will discover a treatment for FM. My reward is the love of my family.

Cybill C. My kids are the driving force that gets me through each day. Sometimes we have beauty hour, when we take turns doing each other's hair and nails. Little things like that mean a lot in a child's mind. My rewards are the good days. They seem to be getting more frequent. Just being able to lie in bed at night and know that I had a good day is reward enough for now.

Patricia S. The most important thing that drives me is my love for my boyfriend. He makes it worthwhile. It really is true that all you need is love. (And money to pay the bills.) Sometimes I feel like my best days are behind me, but life keeps surprising me and remaining interesting.

▲▲▲

Around the time I was diagnosed, two family members passed on, one from colon cancer and one from AIDS. They were a mother and a son, two treasured people whom I miss very much. A family member said to me, "At least you don't have cancer or AIDS." At the time, I was saddened by the comment because I knew the speaker didn't fully understand the pain of FM. I wasn't feeling sorry for myself; I just wanted my family to "get it." Since then I have educated my family, and now they know how FM has changed my life. In some ways, I agree with the relative who made the comment: AIDS, cancer, MS, and lupus are progressive, debilitating illnesses that I am lucky not to have.

Around the same time, a guest speaker at my support group announced that she had terminal cancer in addition to her FM. She urged us to get each of our symptoms checked, rather than lumping them together as "just another FM symptom; I don't need to tell the doctor about it." She told our group that she put off telling her doctor about the blood in her stools, and it turned out to be cancer.

Those two moments were life-changing for me. My family members and I were all sick at once, and now two are gone. My lesson in that was, yes, I have FM, but it's not my whole life, even though it has changed me in every important way. So what keeps me going is the fact that I can.

GOALS

Each of us had goals before fibromyalgia entered our lives. I wanted to manage a flower shop, purchase a home, settle into my new relationship. I wanted to buy every beautiful piece of antique furniture I could afford. Some of these things came to pass, showing me that with or without a chronic illness, even living life in the slow lane, I can accomplish the things I want.

Cybill C. I had many long-term and short-term goals prior to getting sick. I planned to travel and to go back to college for a higher degree. I also planned with my husband to have another baby. All those plans have changed to accommodate my illness. My only goal is to achieve the highest level of functioning that I can.

Lindamarie M. My goals before were to be happy in my marriage, to be a makeup artist, and to be a successful owner/manager of a beauty salon. Today, my goals are to pray daily to God, to keep humble in all my experiences, and to help others.

Patricia S. My goals before the illness took hold were vague. Just to work until I retired, to continue enjoying my hobbies, and to find a man whom I loved and who shared my lifestyle. After my illness, my goals became to keep the man I love (something very difficult to do with this disease) and to get better. I don't have any long-range goals, as I feel I've accomplished a lot. I just want to feel well again and to have sex. Trying to keep up with my boyfriend, taking care of myself, and keeping abreast of research takes all the energy I have.

Donna P. My goals before my diagnosis were to put every ounce of energy and strength into being the best mother, wife, homemaker, and person I could be. I still believe I'm doing my best, considering, but the quality and quantity of my energy and strength have, of course, been drastically reduced, much to my discouragement. It's sometimes hard to avoid comparing apples to oranges—that is, to compare the great health and high level of involvement I formerly enjoyed to my present state of poor health and reduced involvement—without experiencing discouragement.

Cydney B. I sure won't be the "corporate suit" in my dream job that I once was. My goal now is to stay mobile and do the things my husband and I wanted to do when we retired, although we've done those things earlier than we expected. I want to be able to play with, pick up, and put up with my grandchildren should I ever have any. I want to stay financially comfortable.

Mary H.-B. I had no goals before. Now I'm very centered in helping others reach their potential and to spread the word about people with this illness who are misunderstood.

Katie G. My goals before my illness were to do well and continue to succeed in my career and continue to enjoy it. I had hoped to own a home and to be married. I wanted to explore the beautiful areas surrounding where I live and to continue to run in road races. Now my focus is on how to make the most of my day in terms of minimizing stress and streamlining my life. My daily goals are to meditate, walk, do my exercises—whatever it takes to keep my health balanced. I find that much of what I do during the day is related directly or indirectly to minimizing pain, keeping my energy level up, and optimizing my health. My goals are to avoid overextending myself and to avoid overreacting or getting stressed by keeping well-rested and organized.

My recent goals include securing Social Security benefits and finalizing a lawsuit that ended in mediation. I now need to figure out where and how to live a fulfilling, constructive life, given my current limitations. Maybe I am doing that already.

Val T. My goal before diagnosis was to continue my education. I wanted to go back to college and further my medical degree and to become a nurse practitioner or a physician's assistant. My true loves are medicine and helping others and learning as much as I can about the field.

My goal now is to help others regain some quality of life from this devastating disease. I will also continue to improve my health. In many ways, I'm actually more healthy now than before diagnosis. I take care of myself better than ever. It was a tough adjustment, as I'd always helped others and offered great advice but never followed it myself. Other goals include remaining very close to my family; time is short and I now take time out to "smell the roses."

I did a lot of soul-searching when I became ill, and I have learned that I'm strong-willed and a fighter, and I never give up. I also learned that I was not invincible; things did and can happen to me. After the shock of illness, I realized that I would do everything I could to improve my life. I still do much research on FM and continue to try new therapies. I've learned to be my own best advocate.

SPIRITUAL CHANGE

Fibromyalgia changes us down to the very core of our being. Before my diagnosis, I never took a moment to stop and reflect about my faith. I wasn't sure I even had one. When my illness stopped me in my tracks, I had time to realize that deep inside I had beliefs. Where did they come from? About eight years ago, when I went to an energy therapist, I began to question what might have happened to me in other lives. I'd always had an interest in spiritual subjects, but I was a solid skeptic. I made this appointment on the advice of a friend. I hadn't met the therapist before. As soon as we began, she told me that someone was with us and went on to describe my family member who'd just died of AIDS. Through her, Bill and I spoke.

This comforted me, and it began my spiritual awakening. Since then, several unexplainable things have happened to me, and I keep my mind open for more.

I believe we become open to the spiritual side of life when our everyday lives are turned upside-down. We find comfort in the rituals of our belief system and lose ourselves and the pain in prayer and meditation.

Cybill C. Spiritually, I have grown so much. I am a firm believer in God. On days when I am well enough, I attend church. The power of prayer is wonderful. I have never felt as close to God as when I got sick. On very bad days, I feel the spirits of loved ones since passed. At first I was afraid, because I thought it meant I was dying soon and they were coming to prepare me. I even made out my living will and last will and testament! But then I realized that they were here to comfort me.

Sonia H.   Before, I was always on such a run, just dashing from one thing to the next, and I never stopped to think about taking time to contemplate or meditate. It was always do, do, do and accomplish and produce. When I was practically bedridden for a while, I certainly had the time to do some reading and some spiritual searching, so in that process I became more willing to put my faith in something. I didn't have to do it all myself. I felt a dependence on the spirit.

Katie G.   FM has deepened my spiritual awareness. I always thought I was spiritual, but this has catapulted it. I realize everyone has a journey to follow, lessons to learn, and hardships to face. Few truly have it easy. Becoming sick at such a young age also forced me to come face-to-face with mortality. Life as we know it doesn't go on forever. The body is vulnerable and things do happen to it.

One night, I was particularly sick with night sweats. I suddenly woke up, drenched from perspiration, and saw two spiritlike, grayish bodies vibrating up and down at the foot of my bed. At first I thought, "Great, I am hallucinating." Then it was as if my mind clicked and I knew one of the spirits was my paternal grandmother, who'd died twenty-one years earlier. In my mind, I called her name and started to cry, saying I was so sick. She responded (telepathically?) that she knew I was and that's why she was there. Boom—I fell back in bed totally at ease and at peace and went back to sleep. It was the briefest encounter. Over the next several days, I tried to discount the event. However, it was as if my grandmother knew I would do so, and she left signs of her presence. I would smell her scent out of the blue. I was blow-drying my hair and smelled the grilled-cheese sandwiches she made for us as children. The scent was so strong I actually turned off the hairdryer and went into the kitchen to make sure nothing was on the stove.

The experience gave me tremendous comfort and joy. I realize she and others are around and that I am never truly alone.

Having FM/CFS does not take away from our spiritual nature—probably only enhances it. We are still spiritual beings, even though the physical part has changed. I find I am more in tune with people and far more intuitive than before.

Cheryl R. I was feeling so bad and so low, I was truly starting to feel lost in myself, and I turned to my heavenly father for the answers to my problems. Still today I find that to be the best thing about this whole situation. I am blessed and very happy. I have learned that if we want others to understand this illness we have to see it from their perspective.

My rewards in this life include anticipation for where I'm going next, knowing that the Lord and my family all love me no matter what. That is what I live for. I never feel alone anymore. I love my Lord!

Victoria M. I have been amazed by the positive outcomes in my life as a consequence of having faith and of asking for help in prayer, which I had not really done before. There is not a day that goes by when I fail to pray and acknowledge my thanks. My spiritual strength was what kept me going. I needed help. I was so devastated and confused by everything that was happening to me and my family that I looked for pure thought and support. By opening myself to prayer, little miracles have occurred.

Rae H. Spirituality is one of the most important components of my life. Prayer and church are crucial to my sense of well-being. I must admit that I've done this in spite of FM. Very early on in my spiritual maturation, I stopped blaming God for the "bad thing" that had happened. Although I feel gratitude for the good things in my life, I don't necessarily "credit" God with bringing them. I think of "God" or "Spirit" as a deep well of support and presence that I can draw strength from, as a source of nurturing and courage. I cannot imagine life having any quality, regardless of my health status, if I didn't have this sense of Spirit in my daily world.

Gina H. Fibromyalgia has made me hit rock bottom. After trying to do the right thing, this is what I get. Yet I am still holding onto that mustard seed. I will be okay. I almost let go because I felt I could not take it anymore. Pain, depression, and problems have had me down. But God stepped in and said don't let go.

I really can't look into the future because life sometimes throws you a lemon. Right now I am living day to day and hoping for a cure. Writing my book is something I do that I look forward to. The name of it is *We Don't Look Sick,* because that's what FM patients hear all the time. Sometimes I feel that God is trying to get me ready for the next chapter. Today I am here because of God's mercy.

Alison H.   Wow, have I learned a lot! I learned that I was not a whole human being—that there were many things out there I had cut myself off from. I learned that I can't be self-reliant and that trusting God will get me through. I learned that to be happy I don't have to be completely healthy, but I have to find love. I have to find the kind of love Jesus had for me. I learned that sometimes you have to give in and rest a little while. I've learned that I'm not sup-posed to be able to do everything, but there are still a lot of things I can do. And I've learned to get the most out of every day because I don't know how many I have left—that's the only way to truly expe-rience joy.

Gerry L.   I recently discovered that I love the millennia-old rituals of my church that began as pagan rituals but are still such a rich and important part of it for me. Expressing my spirituality has become very emotional for me. There was a time when it was diffi-cult to go to mass. It was painful, the tears would flow, and my husband had a hard time seeing me that way.

I also love walking and noticing nature, walking a labyrinth, and exploring chakras, karma, and chi (life-force energy). I'm comfort-able knowing that going to a Buddhist temple was the right thing for me to do for a time.

Nancy D.   My spirituality was well-established because I was once fortunate enough to be married to an alcoholic, and through his recovery efforts I also found group and educational support. Those meetings are where I discovered the power of attending a supportive meeting to teach me how to live. I found the FM/CFS support groups to be inspirational, and I got reminded many times that there are angels here on earth.

▲▲▲

OTHER WAYS WE'VE CHANGED

My therapist told me of a study about the power of words. A scientist who grew rock crystals in jars taped words on the outside of the jars. The rock crystals in jars labeled with words such as *love* or *peace* flourished. The rock crystals in jars labeled *hate* or *poison* didn't grow or were stunted. Similarly, my sister-in-law says that if she reminds my brother, "Don't forget to empty the dishwasher," he will forget to do it. If she tells him, "Remember to empty the dishwasher," by golly, it's empty when she comes home.

I have changed my language from the negative self-talk I learned in my younger years. Now I pepper my sentences and thoughts with positive words and phrases. I will not use the word *can't*. *Can't* means I'm back at three years old and I "can't have" whatever it is I want. It's a self-defeating word. And there are much better words out there, such as "I choose not to." Try it; it works. This is another example of a big change I've created by making a few small changes.

Sisu G. You find out that the person you thought you were has nothing on the person you really are. Even when I put all of my energy into appearing normal so that I can have a somewhat normal life, I still somehow have enough energy left to believe that this is not the end of me.

I'm now much more aware that the things we use as measurements of worth—wealth, ability, career—all can be interrupted and still leave the essential person untouched. If that's the case, how can they be accurate measures? I never even realized that I used them, never knew that I was trying to live up to them until I couldn't anymore. Now I've had to find my self-worth in other places, and I've found other people's there as well.

Rachel B. I think my relationship with my partner has become closer. Whenever something is helping me, we find a sense of joy and hope. During the times when we are both down, we try to find humor in the situation.

Val T. My family members and I are all much stronger and closer than before. I had to accept help and to quit being so independent, so this illness became a positive thing that brought us all closer. I've also found a new willingness to help others. Simply giving a little ray of hope to someone may save a life. I'm a much stronger person than ever before. I feel proud of my accomplishments since diagnosis. I nearly died several months ago, and even though it was terrifying for me and my family, good things came out of it! My thoughts and feelings have changed for the better, and I have new meaning to my life. I no longer take it for granted.

Sondra H. I've learned that I'm a survivor and a fighter. That I could come from such a low place and rebuild my life in an altered fashion makes me feel so blessed. I appreciate everything so much more. The illness has changed me mentally and spiritually; it has made me look inside myself. A lot of times, as mothers and wives, we give and give and never think much about ourselves. But having FM has made me stop and discover some very deep places within myself.

Penny G. I feel great gratitude for the beauty in nature that I now have time to enjoy. I have forgiven myself for not being perfect. I have found out who my loving, caring friends really are. I have a closer relationship with my husband and daughter, because I really need them now.

Katie G. Some people have told me how they admire the fact that I have not stopped living or crawled into a hole because of this illness. Comments have been positive about how I have built a life around what I am able to do and to push on ahead without giving up. Through this illness I have been able to pass on to others what has helped me.

Because I have been forced to slow down, I also appreciate life's smaller gifts that I may have failed to notice before. I am very aware of nature—the changing sky, clouds, light, the trees, the birds, the colors. I am grateful when things go easily and I accomplish what I need to. I have grown and appreciate the quiet, the stillness. I can focus much more easily.

In describing her life with FM, below, Suzan expresses so beautifully what many of us have experienced: That having this illness has taught us more than we could have imagined and altered us in ways we may never have expected or wanted. That undergoing those lessons and those changes can seem like walking through fire. That acceptance—of our illness and of our forever modified lives—is a huge part of the healing process. And that gifts sometimes come in strange packages.

Suzan B. People ask me how I've survived the drastic changes in my life. To find peace within my illness I had to admit that my old life was over. That was the hardest thing. I tried to retain all I could of my previous life, but as soon as I let go, I was able to start anew. I have a new life now. I am a different person. Few people get the chance to rebuild themselves. I had no choice, but I must say it has been good for me. I am a much different, much better person now than ever before. The illness has been a teacher for me.

When I first got sick, I lost everything. I lost my identity. If I was no longer a biotechnology microbiologist and white-water raft guide, who was I? I had to accept that I was no longer a strong, independent person who never had to ask for help with anything and who was used to taking care of others. I had done all of my own car repairs and maintenance. I ran several times a week; I worked out with weights and was stronger than most men. I made most of the gifts I gave others out of stained glass. All of that was gone one day when my illness struck. Within the first three months of its onset, I lost my career, my health, my independence, my apartment, my boyfriend, my pet rabbit, and my great love: white-water rafting.

All of those activities had defined my life and who I was in the world. Now, activity could no longer define me. I felt like a blank slate. It took me a while to realize that I had to begin writing on it anew. I began questioning my values. My old values centered around money and job status. I started asking myself, "What is really important?" I soon decided that there is nothing more important than people and how we treat each other. I realized that who I am is more important than what I do.

I started tapping into my spiritual side, in spite of my previous extreme resistance to anything related to a church. I even started going to church, and once I regained some ability to read, I began reading spiritual books. My motto became "Get spiritual or die" as I searched for meaning in an illness of pain and suffering. I began meditating after my support group took a survey and found it was the one thing that helped people the most consistently across the board. I learned from one minister that we are all so interconnected that even my own personal growth helped others. I nurtured friendships formed through my church and support groups. I found new purpose in supporting others through hard times. I relearned how to laugh. I began collecting board games that make people laugh and invited people over for "laughing parties." I gave out token gifts to the one who laughed the most. I began to learn how to laugh at myself. And I learned survival tools and how to ask for help. That was one of the most difficult lessons of this illness for me. Before my laughing parties I would ask for volunteers to help set up beforehand and clean up afterward. I learned that asking for help can be a gift to others—that just as helping people adds value to my life, so it does the same for others.

Now one of the most important things I do on a daily basis is to keep my spirits up. This is a spiritual practice, and spiritual practices are best done on a daily basis. Things I do include listening to inspiring, upbeat music. Music that touches my soul. Music that I can sing along to at the top of my lungs when I am upset. Music that lifts my spirit. Prayer and meditation keep me in touch with the idea that there is a higher plan here, whether I understand it or not. There is purpose in this illness, as there is purpose in everything. I talk to people on a daily basis. I keep books around that contain short uplifting phrases or sentences, so I can easily and quickly locate an uplifting thought for the day.

I try to use my creativity. When I got sick and lost the function of my left brain (analytical), I decided that I was supposed to be using my right brain (creative, feeling). Being creative puts me into another state of mind that takes my thoughts off of my life for a while. I might get out my crayons and scribble on large sheets of paper to express my pain and fears in colors. Afterward I feel washed clean of stagnant feelings.

Some people believe that God (Spirit, whatever) gives us all that is good and none of the things we regard as bad. I believe that God has a different viewpoint from ours. I believe God gave me this illness because he/she believes it is a good thing for me. I used to think that I must be able to carry out my life purpose even while I am sick, because otherwise I wouldn't have gotten sick. Now I believe that I got sick in order to fulfill my life purpose. I don't believe I could have fulfilled it if I had continued on the path I was on. I had never really reviewed my values or wondered what will matter to me most when I am on my deathbed, or afterward. That way of life seemed great at the time, but it was lacking in many things—things that weren't important to me then, but that I now see as much more important than anything I was doing. Spirituality is one of those things; another is my relationships with people around me. These have deepened and gained meaning I never experienced before. I have compassion that I could not have acquired through a life of ease. (I've heard many Christians say that all of their saints went through lives of difficulty before their sainthood.) I credit my illness with all of these positive, if hard-won, life changes.

IN CLOSING

I once read a recipe for a "Turpentine Bath for Rheumatic Pains" in a hundred-year-old book about taking care of oneself. The recipe required making an emulsion of black soap and turpentine, shaking it up vigorously until it was "beautiful and creamy," and using it in the bath. It recommended remaining in the bath for forty-five minutes, then wrapping up and getting into bed. When a "prickly sensation" was felt all over the body, the recipe said, the user should take a nap. Afterward, the user should notice a "marked diminution" in the rheumatism pains.

Wow! It sounds about as good as anything else I'm doing these days. It just goes to show how much things have changed in health care—and also how little things have changed. We still don't have a cure for FM, and a hot soak and a nap nearly always help.

To women living with fibromyalgia, I say this: Take the best care of yourself that you can. You are worth the effort. Don't get discouraged when people fail to understand FM. Offer them a little education on the subject, and then let it go. You have done your best. In your heart of hearts, you know that the illness exists and that you are fighting the good fight to get better.

Try some of the everyday solutions we have mentioned in this book, and come up with some of your own. Making your life easier is a top priority.

Love your family and friends just as you always have. You can still have a life; it's just a slower-paced life.

Get the best doctor you can on your side, and keep up your education on this illness. Together, you and your doctor make a terrific team!

Remember Dharma Singh Khalsa's teaching that pain and suffering do not go hand in hand. Focusing on what you don't have and what you might be missing out on, coupled with the very real pain and fatigue of FM, can make your life unbearable.

Yes, we've changed. We have FM to deal with now. But it's only one part of our precious lives. If we remember that, we have won.

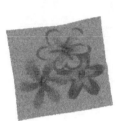

Resources

Glossary

Index

Resources

Fibromyalgia Organizations

Fibromyalgia Network
PO Box 31750
Tucson AZ 85751-1750
(800) 853-2929
Website: www.fmnetnews.com
Subscribers to the FM Network's quarterly newsletter receive a free listing of health-care providers and support groups in their region.

National Fibromyalgia Partnership, Inc.
140 Zinn Way
Linden VA 22642-5609
(866) 725-4404
Fax (toll free): (866) 666-2727
E-mail: mail@fmpartnership.org
Website: www.fmpartnership.org
The website offers many resources, including overviews of lesser-known books from small/independent publishers.

National Fibromyalgia Research Association
PO Box 500
Salem OR 97308
Website: www.nfra.org
NFRA is an advocacy group for FM education and research and a resource for FM patients. The website provides links to articles, educational material, and other FM organizations.

Oregon Fibromyalgia Foundation (OFF)
1221 SW Yamhill, Ste. 303
Portland OR 97205
Voice mail: (503) 892-8811

Website: www.myalgia.com
OFF was founded by prominent FM researcher Dr. Robert Bennett and exercise physiologist Dr. Sharon Clark, both of Oregon Health & Science University. The website offers many resources, including exercise videos produced specifically for the FM patient.

Other Useful Organizations

American Association of Naturopathic Physicians
8201 Greensboro Dr., Ste. 300
McLean VA 22102
(877) 969-2267
(703) 610-9037
Fax: (703) 610-9005
Website: www.naturopathic.org
Website includes a listing of practitioners nationwide.

American Chiropractic Association
1701 Clarendon Blvd.
Arlington VA 22209
(800) 986-4636
Fax: (703) 243-2593
Website: www.amerchiro.org
Website includes a nationwide directory of chiropractors.

American Chronic Pain Association
PO Box 850
Rocklin CA 95677
(800) 533-3231
Website: www.theacpa.org
Online catalog sells audiotapes and CDs to help with relaxation, breathing for pain control, and creating affirmations.

American College of Rheumatology
1800 Century Pl., Ste. 250
Atlanta GA 30345
(404) 633-3777
Fax: (404) 633-1870

E-mail: acr@rheumatology.org
Website: www.rheumatology.org
Website includes a directory of rheumatologists by location.

Arthritis Foundation
PO Box 7669
Atlanta GA 30357-0669
(404) 872-7100
Question-and-answer line (toll free): (800) 283-7800
Website: www.arthritis.org
Call to locate a fibromyalgia support group near you. Website
includes a directory of local foundation chapters, organized by state.

Feldenkrais Guild of North America
3611 SW Hood Ave., Ste. 100
Portland OR 97201
(800) 775-2118
(503) 221-6612
Fax: (503) 221-6616
Website: www.feldenkrais.com
Call or visit the website to locate a Feldenkrais practitioner in your
area.

Social Security Administration
Office of Public Inquiries
Windsor Park Building
6401 Security Blvd.
Baltimore MD 21235
(800) 772-1213
Website: www.ssa.gov
To locate the Social Security Administration office nearest you, call
or visit the website. The website also offers extensive services and
information, including an online application for Social Security disability benefits.

Websites

www.ImmuneSupport.com Operated by Pro Health, Inc., this site provides links to over three thousand articles and abstracts on FM and CFS. It also features a FM/CFS message board, a chat room, a "good doctor list," and links to other FM/CFS resources. The site is updated every two to three days with coverage of new research, treatments, and interviews with top researchers.

www.fmscommunity.org One of the original online resources for FM'ers, the Fibromyalgia Community website offers an online newsletter, links to the subscriber-only mailing list Fibrom-L Listserv, book reviews, fibromyalgia-friendly products, and many other resources.

www.WebMD.com A comprehensive health-care website, WebMD includes a search feature linking users to information on many health conditions. Also offers message boards and "online communities," some with professional moderators, specific to many conditions.

www.disabilityadvocates.com Disability Advocates is an organization of nonattorney representatives that provides legal services to clients seeking Social Security disability benefits. Although the firm is a for-profit business, its website offers much good information about the process involved in obtaining Social Security benefits.

Newsletters

Fibromyalgia Frontiers
Published by the National Fibromyalgia Partnership, Inc., for its members.
(For contact information, see "Fibromyalgia Organizations," above.)

The Fibromyalgia Network Newsletter
Published by the Fibromyalgia Network
(For contact information, see "Fibromyalgia Organizations," above.)

Health Points
Published by To Your Health, Inc.
17007 East Colony Dr., #106
Fountain Hills AZ 85268
(800) 801-1406
Website: www.e-tyh.com
National newsletter advocating complementary therapies, with a focus on FM, CFIDS, arthritis, and chronic pain.

Healthwatch
Published by Pro Health, Inc.
(For contact information, see "Products and Practitioners," below.)

INFA News
Published by the Inland Northwest Fibromyalgia Association
3021 S. Regal, #103
Spokane WA 99223
(509) 838-3001
Fax: (509) 838-8656
E-mail: info@spokanefm.org
Website: www.spokanefm.org

Practitioners and Products

Energy Therapy
Marti MacEwan, M.A., L.M.H.C.
(206) 362-8167
E-mail: marti@energytherapist.com
Website: www.energytherapist.com
The website includes detailed information about energy therapy (see Chapter 12). It also provides links to other websites that list energy therapists nationwide.

FM Exercise Video
By exercise physiologist Sharon Clark, Ph.D., F.N.P.
Oregon Fibromyalgia Foundation
(For contact information, see "Fibromyalgia Organizations," above.)

Updated video includes segments on stretching, relaxation, and education, specifically designed for the FM patient.

Gravity Werks
Eduardo Barrera
3272 California Ave SW, Seattle WA 98116
(206) 933-1411
Gravity Werks uses Thomas Hanna's Somatics Education and Geoff Gluckman's Muscle Balance and Function Development to work with the whole body in order to promote wellness and ease of movement. Audiotapes of Ed Barrera's somatics programs (see Chapter 5) are available from Gravity Werks.

Pro Health, Inc.
2040 Alameda Padre Serra, Ste. 101
Santa Barbara CA 93103
(800) 366-6056
Fax: (805) 965-0042
E-mail: customerservice@prohealthinc.com
Website: www.prohealthinc.com
Pro Health is the largest retailer of FM- and CFS-focused health products, including dietary supplements, the Alpha Stim microcurrent unit, and the Cuddle Ewe line of wool-batting bed accessories.

Schwan's
Website: www.schwans.com
Schwan's delivers frozen meals to many locations throughout the United States. Orders can be placed on the website.

Further Reading

Armitage, Kathleen J., M.D. *The ABC Workbook of Fibromanagement for Fibromyalgia*. Brampton, Ontario: Brampton Rehabilitation, Inc., 2000. (To order, call (905) 455-4088, or visit Dr. Armitage's website at www.fibromanagement.com.)

Berne, Katrina, Ph.D. *Chronic Fatigue Syndrome, Fibromyalgia, and Other Invisible Illnesses: A Comprehensive and Compassionate Guide* (formerly *Running On Empty*). Alameda, CA: Hunter House, 2002.

Bigelow, Stacie. *Fibromyalgia: Simple Relief Through Movement.* New York: John Wiley and Sons, 2000.

Golan, Ralph, M.D. *Optimal Wellness.* New York: Ballantine Books, 1995.

Hammerly, Milton, M.D. *Fibromyalgia: The New Integrative Approach: How to Combine the Best of Traditional and Alternative Therapies.* Holbrook, MA: Adams Media, 2000.

Prudden, Bonnie. *Myotherapy: Bonnie Prudden's Complete Guide to Pain-Free Living.* New York: Dial Press, 1984.

Singh Khalsa, Dharma, M.D., with Cameron Stauth. *The Pain Cure: The Proven Medical Program That Helps End Your Chronic Pain.* New York: Warner Books, 1999.

Skelly, Mari. *Alternative Treatments for Fibromyalgia and Chronic Fatigue Syndrome: Insights from Practitioners and Patients.* Alameda, CA: Hunter House, 1999.

St. Amand, R. Paul, and Claudia Craig Marek. *What Your Doctor May Not Tell You about Fibromyalgia: The Revolutionary Treatment That Can Reverse the Disease.* New York: Warner Books, 1999.

Starlanyl, Devin J., and Mary Ellen Copeland. *Fibromyalgia and Chronic Myofascial Pain: A Survival Manual* (2nd ed.). Oakland, CA: New Harbinger, 2001.

Starlanyl, Devin J. *The Fibromyalgia Advocate: Getting the Support You Need to Cope with Fibromyalgia and Myofascial Pain Syndrome.* Oakland, CA: New Harbinger, 1998.

Teitelbaum, Jacob, M.D. *From Fatigued to Fantastic: A Proven Program to Regain Vital Health, Based on a New Scientific Study Showing Effective Treatment for Chronic Fatigue and Fibromyalgia* (updated ed.). New York: Avery Penguin Putnam, 2001.

Torkelson, Charlene. *Get Fit While You Sit: Easy Workouts from Your Chair.* Alameda, CA: Hunter House, 1999.

Williamson, Miryam Ehrlich. *The Fibromyalgia Relief Book: 213 Ideas for Improving Your Quality of Life.* New York: Walker and Company, 1998.

Glossary

acupuncture—A diagnostic system used to treat illness, manage chronic disorders, and alleviate pain. It involves the insertion of needles (sometimes combined with the application of heat or electrical stimulation) at precise points on the body. Part of traditional Chinese medicine, acupuncture promotes health through prevention and maintenance, encourages healing, and improves functioning. Chinese medicine, the most widely used healing system in the world, combines acupuncture, herbs, cupping, moxabustion (burning the herb moxa to add heat to the body), massage, diet, and gentle exercise to correct energy imbalances in the body.

acute—Describes a disease or condition with a rapid onset and a short, severe course.

Alexander Technique—A movement therapy that teaches students improved use of the body and helps to identify and change poor or inefficient physical habits that may cause stress or fatigue. This system of physical retraining uses a series of simple movements that put the body into a state of balance and relaxation and encourages students to develop awareness and control in their daily activities. See also *Feldenkrais Method*.

arthritis—Inflammation of a joint, which may cause swelling, redness, and pain. Arthritis is part of the category of rheumatic diseases, in which there is an inflammatory condition involving the joints. (The broader term *rheumatic disease* refers to conditions in which there are changes in connective tissues, including muscles, tendons, joints, bursae, and fibrous tissues.) The two main types of arthritis are *rheumatoid arthritis*, an autoimmune disease, and *osteoarthritis*, also called *degenerative joint disease*.

autoimmune disease—A disorder associated with the body's production of antibodies directed against its own tissues. It can be organ specific, such as Hashimoto's disease (which affects the thyroid), or systemic, such as systemic lupus erythematosus. Rheumatoid arthritis is an autoimmune disease.

biofeedback—A system that trains the mind to gain voluntary control over autonomic body functions. Its goal is to help the patient use enhanced muscle awareness to develop better muscle utilization and release skills.

candida—A complex medical syndrome caused by chronic overgrowth of the yeast *Candida albicans* in body tissues. General symptoms include chronic fatigue, loss of energy, general malaise, and decreased libido. Symptoms may be similar to those of FM and CFS. Most affected are the body's gastrointestinal system (bloating, gas, intestinal cramps, rectal itching, and altered bowel function), endocrine system (primarily menstrual complaints), nervous system (depression, irritability, and inability to concentrate), and immune system (allergies, chemical sensitivities, and low immune function). Treatment includes a low-carbohydrate diet, *Lactobacillus acidophilus* (to promote normal floral growth in the gut), and antifungal medications. Major causes include use of antibiotics, birth control pills, steroids, or immune-suppressing drugs.

chi—The vital life energy believed by practitioners of Asian medicine to flow through the body's acupuncture meridians; known as *qi* in Japanese acupuncture and *prana* in Ayurvedic medicine.

Chinese medicine—A system of medical treatment, thought, and practice developed over two millennia, its therapeutics include acupuncture, herbs, nutrition, massage, and movement techniques such as tai chi.

chiropractic—A health-care system that deals with the relationship between the spinal column and the nervous system. Its philosophy teaches that nerve impulses must flow in an unobstructed manner from the spinal nerves to all parts of the body in order for a person to enjoy harmony, vitality, and good health. It is the most widespread drugless, nonsurgical health system in the Western world.

chronic—Of long duration; used to describe a disease or condition that progresses slowly and lasts more than six months.

chronic fatigue syndrome (CFS)—A specific illness characterized by severe, persistent fatigue, often associated with difficulties of sleep and concentration, aching muscles and joints, headaches, sore throat, and depression. In clinical populations, it is most commonly diagnosed in previously healthy women between the ages of twenty and fifty, but it can afflict people of all ages and socioeconomic groups throughout the world. Also known as *chronic fatigue and immune dysfunction syndrome* (CFIDS).

cognition—Awareness and perception of reality, including all aspects of perceiving, thinking, and remembering.

craniosacral therapy—A gentle, noninvasive, hands-on manipulative technique that helps to detect and correct imbalances in the body's craniosacral system, which can cause various sensory, motor, or intellectual dysfunctions. The craniosacral system is comprised of the brain, spinal cord, cerebrospinal fluid, cranial dural membrane, cranial bones, and sacrum. This therapy is used by many health-care practitioners, including medical doctors, dentists, chiropractors, osteopaths, naturopaths, acupuncturists, and licensed body workers.

debilitating—Leading to limited ability; causing a loss of strength or energy.

diagnosis—The act or process of identifying or determining the nature or cause of a disease or injury through evaluation of patient history and examination and review of laboratory data; also refers to the opinion that results from such evaluation.

Eastern medicine—A term used to refer to non-Western systems of medicine. See also *acupuncture* and *Chinese medicine*.

energy therapy—A treatment approach combining psychotherapy with techniques to correct and heal the body's electromagnetic energy systems. It aims to reduce emotional distress and restore emotional well-being by clearing disturbances in the same energy systems treated in Eastern therapeutic practices such as acupuncture.

Feldenkrais Method—A movement technique focused on body/mind integration that uses movement to enhance communication between the brain and body. Lessons, either one-on-one or in a group, seek to improve students' awareness along with their physical and mental performance. The practitioner guides the student through a series of precise movements that alter habitual patterns and provide new learning directly to the neuromuscular system. Lessons are usually done on a padded table with the student fully clothed.

fibromyalgia (FM)—According to the American College of Rheumatology, FM is a condition diagnosed by chronic, generalized aching in all four quadrants of the body and lasting at least three months, plus the finding, upon physical exam, of pain in at least eleven out of eighteen "tender points" (see below). These sites are more tender than other points in the body.

growth hormone—A substance that stimulates growth and the development of body tissues; specifically, a secretion of the anterior lobe of the pituitary gland that directly influences protein, carbohydrate, and lipid metabolism and controls the rate of skeletal and visceral growth.

Hashimoto's disease—An autoimmune disorder of the thyroid gland in which antibodies are produced against thyroid tissues; most common in middle-aged women. Treatment is administration of thyroid hormones (see also *hypothyroidism*).

heal—To restore to health, balance, or soundness; to cure.

holistic medicine—A form of therapy aimed at treating the whole person, not just the body part or parts in which a symptom occurs; the term refers to the whole body or to the body/mind/spirit connection.

homeopathic/homeopathy—A system of medicine based on the concept that "like cures like." Its basic premise maintains that any substance capable of producing symptoms in a healthy person can cure those symptoms in a sick person. Homeopathic reme-

dies are diluted agents or substances that assist the body in utilizing its own energy to regain balance and health and are derived
from a variety of plant, mineral, and chemical substances.
Homeopathic treatment addresses the patient's entire body and
personality and does not focus solely upon the patient's specific
disease or symptom.

hyperthyroidism—A condition of excessive functional activity of the
thyroid gland. It occurs most commonly as part of a syndrome
that may include enlarged thyroid (goiter) and abnormal protru-
sion of the eyes (exophthalmia). Also known as Grave's disease.

hypnotherapy—A therapy using hypnosis; especially useful for management of chronic pain.

hypothyroidism—A deficiency of thyroid gland activity with under-
production of the hormone thyroxine. In its severe form, it is
called *myxedema* and is characterized by physical and mental
sluggishness, loss of hair, weight gain, cold intolerance, skin
coarsening, mental dulling, fatigue, and menstrual irregularities.
Treatment is administration of thyroid hormones.

irritable bladder syndrome—Also known as *interstitial cystitis*; it is
characterized by increased frequency of contractions in the uri-
nary bladder, associated with an increased need to urinate.

irritable bowel syndrome (IBS)—A group of symptoms that comprises
the most common disorder presented by patients seeking a gas-
troenterologist. Symptoms include altered bowel habits, with
diarrhea, constipation, or both; abdominal pain, gas, and bloating; and an absence of any other detectable organic disease. It is
frequently treated with a high-fiber diet and Bentyl, an antispas-
modic, for pain.

magnetic resonance imaging (MRI)—A diagnostic test used by physicians to view the body's internal tissues and organs.

massage therapy—The manipulation of soft tissue for therapeutic
purposes, either by hand or with a mechanical or electrical appa-
ratus. The use of touch to soothe or gain some degree of relief
from pain is a universal human technique. Specific techniques
include myofascial release therapy, Swedish massage, Rolfing,

Hellerwork, and movement-based techniques such as the Feldenkrais Method and Alexander technique.

multiple chemical sensitivity (MCS)—A term that, like "environmental illness," describes states of ill health caused by exposure to substances normally present in the environment, including foods, molds, pollens, and dusts, as well as chemicals, that do not normally make otherwise healthy people ill. The affected person becomes hypersensitized to these substances, causing the immune system to overreact. MCS symptoms can affect any bodily system and may include headaches, nausea, fatigue, dizziness, confusion, muscle weakness, depression, anxiety, and many other physical and emotional reactions.

Muscle Balance and Function (MBF) program—A system focused on postural realignment that applies a progression of properly sequenced, individualized exercises to restore function to the body. The program's evaluation process reveals muscular imbalances that cause postural misalignment, compensated motion, and injury.

myofascial release therapy—The prefix *myo-* means *muscle*. Myofascial release is a hands-on technique used by therapists to relieve soft tissue (muscle) from the grip of abnormally tight fascia (connective tissue). It is a mild and gentle form of stretching that is used to relieve pain and improve physical function.

naturopathic medicine—A system of holistic and nontoxic approaches to medical therapy, with a strong emphasis on disease prevention and wellness optimization. A licensed naturopathic physician attends a four-year, graduate-level naturopathic medical school and is educated in all the same basic sciences as a medical doctor while also studying naturopathic techniques. Therapeutics include clinical nutrition, acupuncture, homeopathic medicine, botanical medicine, psychology, and lifestyle counseling.

neurology—The branch of health science that deals with the nervous system, both normal and diseased. A neurologist is a specialist in the treatment of neurological diseases.

neurotransmitters—Substances that are released from a neuron and travel along the neuron path to either excite (turn on) or inhibit (turn off) a target cell in the central nervous system (see also *serotonin*). These substances modify or transmit nerve impulses.

nutrition—The process by which a living organism assimilates food and uses it for growth, liberation of energy, and replacement of lost cells. The stages include mastication, digestion, absorption, assimilation, and excretion. Nutrition is the science or study that deals with human food and nourishment. A nutritionist is a specialist in the study and application of nutrition theory.

opioids—Opioids are drugs that mimic the activity of opiate drugs, which are named after their natural source, the opium poppy. The poppy contains several active chemicals, including the opiates morphine and codeine. Synthetically produced opioids include meperidine and methadone. These drugs bind to opiate receptors in the central nervous system and spur the release of endorphins, painkillers, and encephalins, the body's natural opiates.

osteopathy—A system of medicine based on the theory that disturbances in the musculoskeletal system affect other body parts and can cause many disorders that can be corrected by various hands-on manipulative techniques used in conjunction with conventional therapeutic procedures. A doctor of osteopathy specializes in, among other things, the use of osteopathic manipulation.

physical therapy—An exercise system aimed at helping the patient avoid abnormal movement patterns and returning them to the highest possible level of function. A physical therapist treats physical dysfunction or injury by the use of therapeutic exercise and the application of modalities intended to restore or facilitate normal body function.

physiology—All the functions of a living organism or any of its parts.

podiatry—A specialized medical field dealing with the care and study of the foot, including its anatomy, pathology, and medical and surgical treatment. A podiatrist is a specialist in the treatment of foot disorders.

psychiatry—A branch of medicine that seeks to treat mental and emotional disorders. A psychiatrist is a physician who specializes in the treatment of such disorders.

psychotherapy—The treatment of mental and emotional disorders through the use of psychological techniques designed to encourage communication of conflicts and insight into problems, with the goals being personality growth and behavioral modification.

rheumatology—The study and treatment of rheumatic diseases. Rheumatism is any of several pathological conditions of the muscles, tendons, joints, bones, or nerves that are characterized by discomfort and disability. Rheumatology is comprised of those conditions that tend to be chronic and involve the musculoskeletal system: joints, tendons, and muscles. Rheumatological conditions include both congenital and inflammatory arthritis; autoimmune diseases that affect joints, connective tissues, and other parts of the body, such as lupus, Sjögren's syndrome, and scleroderma; and conditions involving chronic pain and muscle pain. A rheumatologist specializes in treating these disorders. The training of a rheumatologist typically lasts two or more years beyond internal medicine training. See also *arthritis*.

serotonin—A hormone and neurotransmitter, 5-hydroxytryptamine (5-HT), that is found in many tissues, including blood platelets, intestinal mucosa, the pineal body, and the central nervous system. It has many functions in the body, including inhibition of gastric secretion, stimulation of smooth muscles, and vasoconstriction. Serotonin has been determined to play a key role in FM and CFS. Because many antidepressants function by modifying how serotonin is used in the body (especially in the central nervous system), they may be prescribed as part of the treatment of FM and CFS.

sleep apnea—A sleep disorder characterized by respiratory interruptions during REM sleep (a stage of sleep characterized by rapid eye movement.) Symptoms include repeated nighttime awakening and excessive daytime sleepiness. It is commonly treated with medications and a continuous positive airway pressure (CPAP) machine, which keeps the body's airway open during sleep.

somatic—Of, relating to, or affecting the physical body, especially as distinguished from the mind or the environment. See also *somatics*, below.

somatics—Thomas Hanna, the originator of Hanna Somatic Education, coined the term "somatics" while he was developing the technique that bears his name. Hanna Somatic Education is a system of neuromuscular education (mind/body training) that aims to free people from pain so they can permanently enjoy more comfortable movement. Educators work with clients to help them develop a more accurate sense of their body and to recondition their muscle control.

syndrome—A group of symptoms that collectively indicate or characterize a disease, psychological disorder, or other abnormal condition.

tai chi—A Chinese system of physical exercises that is based on principles of rhythmic movement, equilibrium of body weight, and effortless breathing and that is designed to build *chi* (vital life energy). Originally developed as a martial art for self-defense, it is characterized by progressing slowly and continuously, without strain, through a sequence of contrasting movements. The objective is to achieve health and tranquillity through movement while developing the mind and body; it teaches students how to control the nervous system in order to put the entire body at rest.

tarsal tunnel syndrome—A symptom complex resulting from compression of the tibial nerve as it passes through the inside of the foot and ankle. It causes a burning, electrical, or tingling pain in the sole of the foot. Symptoms are usually aggravated by walking, exercise, or prolonged standing in one place.

temporomandibular joint syndrome (TMJS)—A dysfunction in which there is a clicking or grinding sensation in the temporomandibular joint; includes pain in or about the ears, tiredness, soreness of the jaw muscle upon waking, and stiffness of the jaw itself. Treatment may include both medical and dental intervention as well as trigger-point and tender-point injections (see below).

tender point—A sensitive, painful area that is sore to the touch and found only in FM patients. There are eighteen such sites in the body; a diagnosis of FM is based upon the finding of at least eleven of these tender points on exam.

thyroid—The largest of the endocrine glands, which produces hormones vital for maintaining normal growth and metabolism. The hormones it secretes are triodothyronine (T3) and tetraiodothyronine (T4). Its disorders include hyperthyroidism, hypothyroidism, Hashimoto's disease, and Wilson's Syndrome (see those glossary entries).

toxin—A poison produced by some plants, animals, pathogenic bacteria, and human activities, such as burning fossil fuels or production of industrial wastes. Exposure to these substances can sometimes be fatal.

trigger point—Differs from the tender points found in FM patients (see above). Part of a specific pain pattern found in myofascial pain syndrome, a trigger point is a hypersensitive area in the myofascia (muscle and connective tissue) that is very painful to the touch. Stimulation of this point also "refers" a sensation of pain to another part of the body.

trigger-point and tender-point injections—The use of various techniques to sedate, desensitize, or eliminate trigger or tender points. By sedating pain in these points, the myofascia are allowed to relax and let the area normalize, which stops the referral of pain to other parts of the body. Anesthetics or saline may be injected, or a dry needle may be inserted.

Western medicine—The system of medicine practiced by most medical doctors in the United States and other parts of the Western world; also known as *conventional medicine* and *allopathic medicine*. It aims to produce relief through drugs, surgery, and other therapeutics.

Wilson's Syndrome—A newly defined hypothyroid condition in which the body is unable to convert inactive hormone into active usable hormone. Treatment is with Cytomel, which contains liothyronine (T3).

yoga—An Indian exercise and movement therapy designed to restore
    harmony, flexibility, and function to the body. Yoga purifies the
    body by releasing toxins and impurities. It works with the
    endocrine system and the nervous system and aligns the spine. It
    brings strength and stamina to the various muscle groups, and
    one of its most important benefits is aiding the digestive system.

Index

ALTERNATIVE TREATMENTS FOR FIBROMYALGIA AND CHRONIC FATIGUE SYNDROME: Insights from Practitioners and Patients *by* Mari Skelly

Many people suffering from FM and CFS are unable to find effective treatment and relief. This book combines interviews with practitioners of alternative therapies—including acupuncture, massage therapy, chiropractic, psychotherapy, and energetic healing—with personal stories from patients. These offer a firsthand look at symptoms; treatments; struggles and successes; lifestyle adaptations and medicine, diet, and activity regimens that might help others. There are also sections on health insurance and Social Security disability.

288 pages ... Paperback $15.95 ... Hardcover $25.95

CHRONIC FATIGUE SYNDROME, FIBROMYALGIA, AND OTHER INVISIBLE ILLNESSES: A Comprehensive and Compassionate Guide *by* Katrina Berne, Ph.D.

A new edition of the classic work *Running on Empty,* this revised and expanded book has the latest findings on chronic fatigue syndrome and comprehensive information about fibromyalgia, a related condition. Related diseases such as environmental illness, breast implant inflammatory syndrome, lupus, Sjögren's syndrome, and postpolio syndrome are also discussed. The book includes possible causes, symptoms, diagnostic processes, and options for treatment.

400 pages ... Paperback $15.95 ... Hardcover $25.95

THE ART OF GETTING WELL: A Five-Step Plan for Maximizing Health When You Have a Chronic Illness
by David Spero, R.N., Foreword by Martin L. Rossman, M.D.

Self-management programs have become a key way for people to deal with chronic illness. In this book, David Spero brings together the medical, psychological, and spiritual aspects of getting well in a five-step approach:

* slow down and use your energy for the things and people that matter
* make small, progressive changes; build self-confidence
* nourish the social ties that are crucial for well-being
* value your body and treat it with affection and respect
* take responsibility for getting the best care you can.

224 pages ... Paperback $15.95 ... Hardcover $25.95

WOMEN LIVING WITH MULTIPLE SCLEROSIS
by Judith Lynn Nichols and Her Online Group of MS Sisters

Judith Nichols was first diagnosed with MS in 1976 and cofounded an online support group of women who helped each other cope with the day-to-day challenges of MS. In this book, members of the group share intimate, emotional accounts of their experiences with MS. Some stories are painful, some are funny, often they are both. The range of deeply personal concerns includes family reactions to the diagnosis, workplace issues, sexuality and spirituality, depression and physical pain, loss of bladder and bowel control, and assistive devices and helpful tools. All topics are discussed freely and frankly, in the way closest friends do.

288 pages ... Paperback $13.95

LIVING BEYOND MULTIPLE SCLEROSIS: A Women's Guide
by Judith Lynn Nichols and Her Online Group of MS Sisters

This sequel to *Women Living with Multiple Sclerosis* focuses on transcending the effects of MS. This book shares the same engaging, conversational tone as the first book. In addition to providing more time-, energy- and sanity-saving techniques, this book talks about ways to live beyond the limitations MS imposes. Topics include the newest treatments for MS and how to maximize their benefits; household accessibility, safety, and remodeling; tips for choosing and using assistive devices; and how to prepare applications for Social Security Disability and insurance benefits.

288 Pages ... Paperback $14.95

WHEN PARKINSON'S STRIKES EARLY: Voices, Choices, Resources and Treatment
by Barbara Blake-Krebs, M.A., & Linda Herman, MLS

This book details the physical, emotional, and social struggles faced by young people with Parkinson's and the roads to self-empowerment that can be found through the support and resources of the PD global community. Topics include the complex array of PD symptoms and the side effects of medications; the unique impact early onset PD has on individuals and society; and current surgery options as described by former patients. The book includes a listing of resources and grassroots advocacy ideas. **All royalties will be donated to PD research.**

288 pages ... Paperback $15.95 ... Hardcover $25.95

To order see last page or call (800) 266-5592

GET FIT WHILE YOU SIT: Easy Workouts from Your Chair
by Charlene Torkelson

Here is a total-body workout that can be done right from your chair, anywhere. It is perfect for office workers, travelers, and those with age-related movement limitations or special conditions. This book offers three programs. The One-Hour Chair Program is a full-body, low-impact workout that includes light aerobics and exercises to be done with or without weights. The 5-Day Short Program features five compact workouts for those short on time. Finally, the Ten-Minute Miracles is a group of easy-to-do exercises perfect for anyone on the go.

160 pages ... 212 b/w photos ... Paperback $12.95 ... Hardcover $22.95

SHAPEWALKING: Six Easy Steps to Your Best Body
by Marilyn Bach, Ph.D., and Lorie Schleck, M.A., P.T.

Millions of Americans want an easy, low-cost approach to total fitness. ShapeWalking is the answer—a program that includes aerobic exercise, strength training, and flexibility stretching and that is suited for exercisers of all levels.

ShapeWalking is ideal for people who want to control weight, develop muscle definition, prevent or reverse loss of bone density, and target-tone the stomach, buttocks, arms, and thighs. This all-new second edition includes over 70 black-and-white photographs as well as updated exercises and resources.

160 pages ... 70 photos ... Paperback $14.95 ... Hardcover $24.95 ... DECEMBER 2002

SELF-HELP FOR HYPERVENTILATION SYNDROME:
Recognizing and Correcting Your Breathing-Pattern
Disorder *by* Dinah Bradley ... 3rd Edition

Chronic hyperventilation especially affects asthmatics, premenstrual and menopausal women, over-achievers, and workaholics. Symptoms include breathlessness, chest pains, palpitations, broken sleep, stomach or bowel problems, dizziness, and anxiety. This book explains causes and symptoms and presents a well-tested program that the author has developed for readers to use in order to break the hyperventilation cycle and breathe freely again.

128 pages ... Paperback $12.95 ... Hardcover $22.95

CHINESE HERBAL MEDICINE MADE EASY: Natural and Effective Remedies for Common Illnesses
by Thomas Richard Joiner

Chinese herbal medicine is an ancient system for maintaining health and prolonging life. This book demystifies the subject by providing clear explanations and easy-to-read alphabetical listings of more than 750 herbal remedies for over 250 common illnesses ranging from acid reflux and AIDS to breast cancer, pain management, sexual dysfunction, and weight loss. Whether you are a newcomer to herbology or a seasoned practitioner, you will find this book to be a valuable addition to your health library.

432 pages ... Paperback $24.95 ... Hardcover $34.95

ANDROGEN DISORDERS IN WOMEN: The Most Neglected Hormone Problem *by* Theresa Cheung

One in ten women in the U.S. suffers from a disorder caused by an imbalance of the so-called male hormones known as androgens. Symptoms may include facial or body hair growth or loss, dull skin, fatigue, and weight gain.

Because doctors tend to dismiss or ignore such symptoms, there has been little information available on androgen disorders—until now. This book discusses the medical and emotional effects that excessive androgens can have, and outlines the various forms of conventional and alternative treatments.

208 pages ... Paperback $13.95 ... Hardcover $23.95

MENOPAUSE WITHOUT MEDICINE
by Linda Ojeda, Ph.D. ... New Fourth Edition

Linda Ojeda broke new ground 15 years ago with this best-selling resource on menopause, giving women a clear understanding of menopausal changes as well as guidelines for effective self-care.

In this new edition she reexamines the hormone therapy debate; suggests natural remedies for depression, hot flashes, sexual changes, and skin and hair problems; and presents an illustrated basic exercise program. She also includes up-to-date information on natural sources of estrogen, including phytoestrogens, and how diet and personality affect mood swings.

352 pages ... 32 illus. ... 62 tables ... Paperback $15.95 ... Hardcover $25.95

To order books see last page or call (800) 266-5592

CREATING EXTRAORDINARY JOY: A Guide to Authenticity, Connection, and Self-Transformation *by* Chris Alexander

Creating Extraordinary Joy takes us on a journey of personal discovery in which we become alive to who we are, where we are in life, and what we value. It also helps us connect to the authenticity and true purpose of others in a condition called "synergy," in which the joining of spirit and emotion between two people creates something greater than both.

Using inspirational teachings, images from nature, simple but powerful exercises, and real-life examples, Chris Alexander describes the ten steps of life mastery. Each step yields a life lesson that takes us toward the goals of deepening our passion, opening to abundance, and giving and receiving love. This inspirational guide is more than a book; it is a pathway to our best self.

288 pages ... Paperback $16.95 ... Hardcover $26.95

THE PLEASURE PRESCRIPTION: To Love, to Work, to Play — Life in the Balance *by* Paul Pearsall, Ph.D.
New York Times Bestseller!

This bestselling book is a prescription for stressed-out lives. Dr. Pearsall maintains that contentment, wellness, and long life can be found by devoting time to family, helping others, and slowing down to savor life's pleasures. Pearsall's unique approach draws from Polynesian wisdom and his own 25 years of psychological and medical research. For readers who have questions about healthy values and balance in their lives, *The Pleasure Prescription* provides the answers.

288 pages ... Paperback $13.95 ... Hardcover $23.95

WRITING FROM WITHIN: A Guide to Creativity and Your Life Story Writing *by* Bernard Selling

Writing from Within has attracted an enthusiastic following among those wishing to write oral histories, life narratives, or autobiographies. Bernard Selling shows new and veteran writers how to free up hidden images and thoughts, employ right-brain visualization, and use language as a way to capture feelings, people, and events. The result is at once a self-help writing workbook and an exciting journey of personal discovery and creation.

320 pages ... Paperback $17.95 ... Third Edition

ORDER FORM

10% DISCOUNT on orders of $50 or more —
20% DISCOUNT on orders of $150 or more —
30% DISCOUNT on orders of $500 or more —
On cost of books for fully prepaid orders

NAME

ADDRESS

CITY/STATE   ZIP/POSTCODE

PHONE   COUNTRY (outside of U.S.)

TITLE	QTY	PRICE	TOTAL
Women Living with Fibromyalgia (paperback)		@ $14.95	
Prices subject to change without notice			

Please list other titles below:

		@ $	
		@ $	
		@ $	
		@ $	
		@ $	
		@ $	
		@ $	
		@ $	

Check here to receive our book catalog ☐   free

Shipping Costs

By Priority Mail: first book $4.50, each additional book $1.00
By UPS and to Canada: first book $5.50, each additional book $1.50
For rush orders and other countries call us at (510) 865-5282

TOTAL _____
Less discount @____% (_____)
TOTAL COST OF BOOKS _____
Calif. residents add sales tax _____
Shipping & handling _____
TOTAL ENCLOSED _____
Please pay in U.S. funds only

☐ Check ☐ Money Order ☐ Visa ☐ MasterCard ☐ Discover

Card # _____ Exp. date _____

Signature _____

Complete and mail to:
Hunter House Inc., Publishers
PO Box 2914, Alameda CA 94501-0914
Website: www.hunterhouse.com
Orders: (800) 266-5592 or email: ordering@hunterhouse.com
Phone (510) 865-5282   Fax (510) 865-4295

WFM 10/2002